Eric A. Coleman, MD, MPH
Editor

Charting a Course
for High Quality
Care Transitions

Charting a Course for High Quality Care Transitions has been co-published simultaneously as *Home Health Care Services Quarterly*®, Volume 26, Number 4 2007.

Pre-publication
REVIEWS,
COMMENTARIES,
EVALUATIONS . . .

"AN EXCELLENT COMPENDIUM OF MAJOR WORK focused on improving care transitions for patients moving from one care setting to another. Whether you are a service provider, researcher or policy maker, you will find in this collection VALUABLE INSIGHTS DRAWN FROM LEADING AUTHORS IN THE CARE TRANSITIONS FIELD. The articles span hospital, home health, and nursing home settings, addressing assessment tools, care models, and performance measures. After reading it, I felt I had been given a whirlwind tour of the care transitions arena. The bibliographies alone are a rich resource! Given the current emphasis throughout care settings on reducing acute care readmissions, Dr. Coleman's monograph makes a significant contribution."

Joanne Handy, RN, MS
President and CEO
Visiting Nurse Association of
Boston and Affiliates

More pre-publication
REVIEWS, COMMENTARIES, EVALUATIONS . . .

"Addresses the challenges, potential solutions, and requirements for a systemic approach to improve quality for patients experiencing transitions in care. . . . Health care professionals, health system administrators, and health plan executives will find USEFUL INFORMATION in the book."

Judith S. Black, MD, MHA
Medical Director of Senior Products, Highmark, an independedent licensee of the Blue Cross and Blue Shield Association

"A TIMELY SURVEY REFLECTING SOME OF THE BEST THINKING IN THIS RAPIDLY EMERGING AREA. An informative discussion of definitions and terminology will help readers appreciate the distinctions among the many and varied approaches being tested to meet the transitions problem. Several chapters deal with special populations such as those with cognitive impairment or those who live in residential care settings. Others address predictors of failed care transitions and measurement of the quality of transitions. The textbook of care transitions cannot yet be written, but this volume PROVIDES A RICH SAMPLING OF THE CURRENT STATE OF KNOWLEDGE, including its large gaps. . . . USEFUL to case managers and discharge planners, to those interested in quality improvement and program design, and to researchers and policy analysts."

Alan Lazaroff, MD
President
Geriatric Medicine Associates
Denver, CO

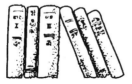

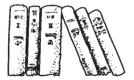

Charting a Course
for High Quality
Care Transitions

Charting a Course for High Quality Care Transitions has been co-published simultaneously as *Home Health Care Services Quarterly*®, Volume 26, Number 4 2007.

Charting a Course for High Quality Care Transitions, edited by Eric A. Coleman, MD, MPH (Vol. 26, No. 4, 2007). *A comprehensive examination of the challenges and opportunities in improving transitional care for older adults.*

Evidence-Based Interventions for Community Dwelling Older Adults, edited by Susan M. Enguídanos, MPH, PhD (Vol. 25, No. 1/2, 2006). *An overview of evidence-based programs that can improve the health of seniors living in community-based settings.*

Improving Medication Management in Home Care: Issues and Solutions, edited by Dennee Frey, PharmD (Vol. 24, No. 1/2, 2005). *A comprehensive examination of the issues and challenges faced in preventing medication errors with effective strategies for managing use in home and community care settings.*

A New Look at Community-Based Respite Programs: Utilization, Satisfaction, and Development, edited by Rhonda J.V. Montgomery, PhD (Vol. 21, No. 3/4, 2002). *"Clear, straightforward, and well focused on practical issues of service delivery . . . maintains a high standard of scholarship. A must-read for anyone interested in planning or evaluating respite services . . . . The first large-scale, longitudinal study of respite use. Service professionals, policymakers, and researchers in health policy, gerontology, and medical sociology will find the text of great value." (Judith G. Gonyea, PhD, Associate Professor, Boston University School of Social Work)*

The Next Generation of AIDS Patients: Service Needs and Vulnerabilities, edited by George J. Huba, PhD, Lisa A. Melchoir, PhD, A. T. Panter, PhD, Vivian B. Brown, PhD, David A. Cherin, PhD, and June Simmons, LCSW (Vol. 19, No. 1/2, 2001). *"Especially interesting in this volume is the presentation of an empirical model (CHAID) that both community-based organizations and service delivery systems can use to analyze client input to monitor and refine their HIV services." (Donna G. Anderson, PhD, MPH, Associate Professor, University of Colorado Health Sciences Center)*

AIDS Capitation, edited by David Alex Cherin, PhD, and G. J. Huba, PhD (Vol. 17, No. 1, 1998). *"A valuable resource to those interested in the blending of curative and palliative care and the application of this blended approach to catastrophic disease management." (Victor L. Kovner, MD, FACP, Medical Director, Sun Alliance Hospice)*

Personal Response Systems: An International Report of a New Home Care Service, edited by Andrew S. Dibner, PhD (Vol. 13, No. 3/4, 1993). *"Does a great service by reporting the forward strides taking place in other nations in the use of personal response systems (PRS)." (Daniel Thursz, DSW, ACSW, President, The National Council of Aging, Inc., Washington, DC)*

Facilitating Self Care Practices in the Elderly, edited by Barbara J. Horn, PhD, RN (Vol. 11, No. 1/2, 1990). *"Useful to researchers, practitioners, caregivers, and agencies providing care services to the elderly ill at home." (The Indian Journal of Social Work)*

Quality Impact of Home Care for the Elderly, edited by Francis G. Caro, PhD, and Arthur E. Blank, PhD (Vol. 9, No. 2/3, 1989). *"An excellent source of information for those wishing to increase their understanding of the home health care system or improve its effectiveness in their own community." (American Journal of Occupational Therapy)*

Worlds Apart?: Long-Term Care in Australia and the United States, edited by Sandra J. Newman, PhD (Vol. 8, No. 3, 1988). *An insightful comparison of how Australia and the United States are responding to the long-term care needs of the elderly.*

Health Care for the Elderly: Regional Responses for National Policy Issues, edited by Kathleen Gainor Andreoli, DSN, Leigh Anne Musser, MPH, and Stanley Joel Reiser, MD, PhD (Vol. 7, No. 3/4, 1987). *"One of the best, most comprehensive, and most penetratingly analytical works on elderly health care now available." (Health and Social Work)*

International Perspectives on Long-Term Care, edited by Laura Reif and Brahna Trager (Vol. 5, No. 3/4, 1985). *Experts from around the world address organizational and cost issues while offering innovative solutions for common problems in long-term care.*

Community-Based Systems of Long-Term Care, edited by Rick T. Zawadski, PhD (Vol. 4, No. 3/4, 1984). *Essential information on planning long-term health care services for the community.*

The Chronically Limited Elderly: The Case for a National Policy for In-Home and Supportive Community-Based Services, edited by Howard A. Palley, PhD, and Julianne S. Oktay, PhD (Vol. 4, No. 2, 1983). *"Compelling reading for those concerned about the non-institutional care of impaired elderly persons." (The Gerontologist)*

Family Home Care: Critical Issues for Services and Policies, edited by Robert Perlman, PhD (Vol. 3, No. 3/4, 1983). *"An important reference for those professionals working in the field of home health care." (Contemporary Sociology)*

Home Health Care and National Health Policy, edited by Brahna Trager (Vol. 1, No. 2, 1980). *A concise study of the current status of home health care in the United States.*

Charting a Course for High Quality Care Transitions

Eric A. Coleman, MD, MPH
Editor

Charting a Course for High Quality Care Transitions has been co-published simultaneously as *Home Health Care Services Quarterly*®, Volume 26, Number 4 2007.

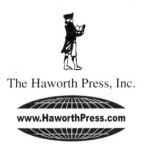

The Haworth Press, Inc.
www.HaworthPress.com

Published by

The Haworth Press, Inc., 10 Alice Street, Binghamton, NY 13904-1580 USA

Charting a Course for High Quality Care Transitions has been co-published simultaneously as *Home Health Care Services Quarterly*®, Volume 26, Number 4 2007.

The development, preparation, and publication of this work has been undertaken with great care. However, the publisher, employees, editors, and agents of The Haworth Press and all imprints of The Haworth Press, Inc., including The Haworth Medical Press® and Pharmaceutical Products Press®, are not responsible for any errors contained herein or for consequences that may ensue from use of materials or information contained in this work. Opinions expressed by the author(s) are not necessarily those of The Haworth Press, Inc. With regard to case studies, identities and circumstances of individuals discussed herein have been changed to protect confidentiality. Any resemblance to actual persons, living or dead, is entirely coincidental.

The Haworth Press is committed to the dissemination of ideas and information according to the highest standards of intellectual freedom and the free exchange of ideas. Statements made and opinions expressed in this publication do not necessarily reflect the views of the Publisher, Directors, management, or staff of The Haworth Press, Inc., or an endorsement by them.

Library of Congress Cataloging-in-Publication Data

Charting A Course for High Quality Care Transitions / Eric A. Coleman, editor.
     p. cm.
     "Co-published simultaneously as Home Health Care Services Quarterly, Volume 26, Number 4 2007."
     Includes bibliographic references and index.
     ISBN-13: 978-0-7890-3742-8 (hard cover : alk paper)
     ISBN-13: 978-0-7890-3743-5 (soft cover : alk. paper)
     1. Home care services–Quality control. 2. Continuum of care–Quality control. I. Coleman, Eric A. II. Home health care services quarterly.
     [DNLM: 1. Home Care Services. 2. Continuity of Patient Care. 3. Models, Theoretical. 4. Patient Care Planning. 5. Quality Assurance, Health Care. 6. Risk Factors. W1 HO502R v.26 no.4 2007 / WY 115 C486 2007]
  RA645.3.C43 2007
  362.14--dc22

                                                2007031713

This section provides you with a list of major indexing & abstracting services and other tools for bibliographic access. That is to say, each service began covering this periodical during the year noted in the right column. Most Websites which are listed below have indicated that they will either post, disseminate, compile, archive, cite or alert their own Website users with research-based content from this work. (This list is as current as the copyright date of this publication.)

Abstracting, Website/Indexing Coverage . . . . Year When Coverage Began

- **Academic Search Premier (EBSCO)****
  <http://search.ebscohost.com> 2006

- **CINAHL (Cumulative Index to Nursing & Allied Health Literature) (EBSCO)**** <http://www.cinahl.com> 1983

- **CINAHL Plus (EBSCO)**** <http://search.ebscohost.com> 2006

- **International Pharmaceutical Abstracts (Thomson Scientific)**** 1991

- **MasterFILE Premier (EBSCO)****
  <http://search.ebscohost.com> 2006

- **MEDLINE (National Library of Medicine)****
  <http://www.nlm.nih.gov> 2000

- **Psychological Abstracts (PsycINFO)****
  <http://www.apa.org> 1985

- **PubMed**** <http://www.ncbi.nlm.nih.gov/pubmed/> 2000

- **Social Services Abstracts (ProQuest CSA) ****
  <http://www.csa.com> 1990

- **Social Work Abstracts (NASW)****
  <http://www.silverplatter.com/catalog/swab.htm> 1982

- **Sociological Abstracts (ProQuest CSA)****
  <http://www.csa.com> 1990

(continued)

(continued)

Bibliographic Access

- ***Cabell's Directory of Publishing Opportunities in Management <http://www.cabells.com/>***

- ***MedBioWorld <http://www.medbioworld.com>***

- ***MediaFinder <http://www.mediafinder.com/>***

- ***Ulrich's Periodicals Directory: The Global Source for Periodicals Information Since 1932 <http://www.bowkerlink.com>***

Special Bibliographic Notes related to special journal issues (separates) and indexing/abstracting:

- indexing/abstracting services in this list will also cover material in any "separate" that is co-published simultaneously with Haworth's special thematic journal issue or DocuSerial. Indexing/abstracting usually covers material at the article/chapter level.
- monographic co-editions are intended for either non-subscribers or libraries which intend to purchase a second copy for their circulating collections.
- monographic co-editions are reported to all jobbers/wholesalers/approval plans. The source journal is listed as the "series" to assist the prevention of duplicate purchasing in the same manner utilized for books-in-series.
- to facilitate user/access services all indexing/abstracting services are encouraged to utilize the co-indexing entry note indicated at the bottom of the first page of each article/chapter/contribution.
- this is intended to assist a library user of any reference tool (whether print, electronic, online, or CD-ROM) to locate the monographic version if the library has purchased this version but not a subscription to the source journal.
- individual articles/chapters in any Haworth publication are also available through the Haworth Document Delivery Service (HDDS).

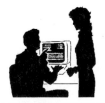

As part of Haworth's continuing commitment to better serve our library patrons, we are proud to be working with the following electronic services:

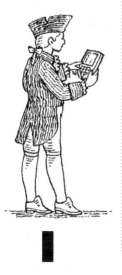

AGGREGATOR SERVICES

EBSCOhost

Ingenta

J-Gate

Minerva

OCLC FirstSearch

Oxmill

SwetsWise

LINK RESOLVER SERVICES

1Cate (Openly Informatics)

ChemPort (American Chemical Society)

CrossRef

Gold Rush (Coalliance)

LInkOut (PubMed)

LINKplus (Atypon)

LinkSolver (Ovid)

LinkSource with A-to-Z (EBSCO)

Resource Linker (Ulrich)

SerialsSolutions (ProQuest)

SFX (Ex Libris)

Sirsi Resolver (SirsiDynix)

Tour (TDnet)

Vlink (Extensity, formerly Geac)

WebBridge (Innovative Interfaces)

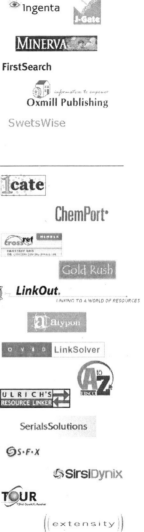

Charting a Course
for High Quality
Care Transitions

CONTENTS

ABOUT THE EDITOR

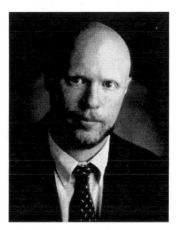

Eric A. Coleman, MD, MPH, is an Associate Professor of Medicine within the Divisions of Health Care Policy and Research and Geriatric Medicine at the University of Colorado at Denver and Health Sciences Center. As a board-certified geriatrician, Dr. Coleman maintains direct patient care responsibility for older adults in ambulatory, acute, and subacute care settings.

Dr. Coleman's research focuses on: (1) enhancing the role of patients and caregivers in improving the quality of their care transitions across acute and post-acute settings; (2) measuring the quality of care transitions from the perspective of patients and caregivers; (3) implementing system-level practice improvement interventions and (4) using health information technology to promote safe and effective care transitions.

Dr. Coleman concurrently pursued his medical degree from the University of California, San Francisco and a Master's in Public Health and Aging from the University of California, Berkeley. He completed residency training in primary care internal medicine, fellowship training in The Robert Wood Johnson Clinical Scholars Program and geriatric medicine at the University of Washington.

Preface

Care Transitions are a time of heightened vulnerability for older adults with complex care needs and ensuring that their needs are met during times of transfer poses a significant challenge. Everyday, hundreds of thousands of older adults transition between affiliated and unaffiliated health care settings, and yet this critical area remains relatively unexplored in the clinical and scientific communities. Fortunately, this trend will dramatically change as the need to improve care coordination across distinct health care settings gains attention from some of the nation's most respected public and private quality oriented organizations. In the past five years, the Institute of Medicine, Joint Commission on Accreditation of Healthcare Organizations, Centers for Medicare and Medicaid Services and its affiliated Home Health Quality Improvement Organization Support Center, Institute for Healthcare Improvement, National Quality Forum, Case Management Society of American, Society for Hospital Medicine, and the American Board of Internal Medicine Foundation have all sponsored national efforts aimed at improving quality during care transitions.

These positive developments will demand that health care providers understand how to overcome the inherent challenges and become equipped with user-friendly tools, care models, and measures to monitor their performance. This special volume of *Home Health Care Services Quarterly*, entitled, "Charting a Course for High Quality Care Transitions" is designed to inform practitioners, quality improvement entities, researchers, and policymakers on effective strategies for ensuring quality and safety at the time of transfer. The title is designed to capture both the early exploratory stage of the field as well as the

[Haworth co-indexing entry note]: "Preface." Coleman, Eric A. Co-published simultaneously in the *Home Health Care Services Quarterly*® (The Haworth Press, Inc.) Vol. 6, No. 1/2, 2007, pp. xxi-xxii; and: *Charting a Course for High Quality Care Transitions* (ed: Eric A. Coleman) The Haworth Press, 2007, pp. xvii-xviii. Single or multiple copies of this article are available for a fee from The Haworth Document Delivery Service [1-800-HAWORTH, 9:00 a.m. - 5:00 p.m. (EST). E-mail address: docdelivery@haworthpress.com].

xvii

importance of making navigational tools readily available for direct application by the practicing clinician.

This sentinel document represents perhaps the most significant collective response to this problem by many of the most prominent leaders in the field. Holland and Harris begin by proposing a practical semantic framework for overcoming one of the most insidious barriers to quality improvement–the lack of a consistent use of terms that define the problem at hand. Rosati and Huang follow with a rigorously developed and tested tool designed to identify home health care patients at risk for hospital readmission that can help home health agencies decide how to best allocate increasingly scarce resources. Using acute stroke as an ideal tracer condition, Kind and colleagues highlight the complex array of medical and social factors that contribute to poor quality care transitions that eventually result in return to high intensity care settings. Next, Naylor and colleagues detail how they plan to extend an Advanced Practice Nurse transitional care model that has proven successful in improving outcomes to the population of cognitively impaired older adults. Parsons and Boling highlight the unique and unrecognized needs of older adults living in residential care facilities. Coleman and colleagues highlight the integral role of patient-centered performance measurement in driving transitional care quality improvement in a "real-world" community hospital setting. Shifting to the national stage, Boyce and Feldman share early results of the Reducing Acute Care Hospitalization National Demonstration Collaborative, comprised of 225 participating home health care agencies. Boling and Parsons conclude this special volume with a look forward, proposing a research agenda designed to identify and fill our knowledge gaps well into the future.

Thus, with so many esteemed national organizations providing a strong tail wind to fill our sails, I invite you aboard this ship with its able-bodied crew as we chart a course for high quality care transitions using practical tools, models, and measures to navigate yet unexplored land and sea.

Eric Coleman, MD, MPH

Introduction

Marian Essey, RN, BSN

Healthcare providers regularly face the challenges of improving the quality of care for patients they serve. Quality may be defined not only as it relates to quality measures for individual provider settings, but also in terms of the quality of care that occurs during care transitions (as patients move from one setting or location to another). These movements or transitions are often unplanned and may occur at the most unforeseen times, such as nights or weekends, when healthcare delivery systems are tested because of staff shortages or busier environments. To complicate matters further, the patient and caregivers are generally ill-prepared for their role in the next care setting. Patient safety can be jeopardized when this situation occurs, and medication mismanagement may also occur. Patients who are cognitively impaired offer an even greater challenge, and are potentially at even higher risk for adverse events occurring as care is transitioned across the continuum.

Since we work in such complex systems, there is generally not a single practitioner who takes the lead in coordinating the patient's care between settings, from the sender to the receiver. Who owns the patient during care transitions–the sending team or receiving team? How can we decrease the probability of adverse events such as medication errors or avoidable hospitalizations? Since there are no standardized measures for publicly-reported care transitions, how can we measure the quality of transitional care?

Marian Essey is Director, Home Health Quality Improvement Organization Support Center, Quality Insights of Pennsylvania, Penn Center West, Bldg 2, Suite 220, Pittsburgh, PA 15276 (E-mail: messey@wvmi.org).

[Haworth co-indexing entry note]: "Introduction." Essey, Marian. Co-published simultaneously in *Home Health Care Services Quarterly*® (The Haworth Press, Inc.) Vol. 26, No. 4, 2007, pp. 1-2; and: *Charting a Course for High Quality Care Transitions* (ed: Eric A. Coleman) The Haworth Press, Inc. 2007, pp. 1-2. Single or multiple copies of this article are available for a fee from The Haworth Document Delivery Service [1-800-HAWORTH, 9:00 a.m. - 5:00 p.m. (EST). E-mail address: docdelivery@haworthpress.com].

Available online at http://hhc.haworthpress.com
doi:10.1300/J027v26n04_01

Providing optimal patient care during transitions has a seemingly endless list of challenges, but there are also many opportunities. Certainly the greatest opportunity is to provide true patient-centered care; care that is respectful and responsive to individual patient preferences, needs, and values and ensures that patient values guide all clinical decisions (Crossing the Quality Chasm: A New System for the 21st Century, http://www.nap.edu/catalog.php?record_id=10027#toc). Providing optimal transitions of care through advancements in research, practice, and data measurement will support the transformation of our nation's health care delivery system.

This issue of *Home Health Care Services Quarterly* highlights the challenges and opportunities related to care transitions. Although challenges occur within every setting, health care providers, patients, and caregivers can be better prepared to meet these challenges. Advancing research into emergent care can provide insights into untapped opportunities for collaboration across systems, including emergent ambulance transport, in long-term care settings and in practices with cognitively impaired older adults who are in need of enhanced transitional care. Healthcare delivery systems can also improve in identifying patients at risk for adverse events during transitions, and then more efficiently determine which resources (such as advance practice nurses, care coaches, or home health staff) to use in order to help reduce or eliminate unfavorable outcomes. Finally, measuring quality of care cannot stop when a patient is discharged from a setting. True quality is measured by the patient, not the setting. The opportunities for providing patient-centered care during care transitions far outweigh the challenges.

NOTE

This material was prepared by Quality Insights of Pennsylvania, the Medicare Quality Improvement Organization Support Center for Home Health, under contract with the Centers for Medicare & Medicaid Services (CMS), an agency of the U.S. Department of Health and Human Services. The contents presented do not necessarily reflect CMS policy. Publication number: 8SOW-PA-HHQ07.371. App: 3/05/07.

Discharge Planning, Transitional Care, Coordination of Care, and Continuity of Care: Clarifying Concepts and Terms from the Hospital Perspective

Diane E. Holland, PhD, RN
Marcelline R. Harris, PhD, RN

SUMMARY. Hospital discharge planning is a key element of continuity of care for persons leaving the hospital. Yet many important questions regarding processes and effects of discharge planning have not been addressed, in part because the multiple terms associated with discharge planning have not been consistently defined or used. Failure to clearly name, define, and consistently use terms creates a barrier that inhibits scientific progress and best practice. This article reviews the use of terms and definitions and compares concepts associated with hospital discharge planning across key documents frequently referenced by hospitals. A conceptual model is proposed to facilitate consistent use of these concepts. doi:10.1300/J027v26n04_02 *[Article copies available for a fee from The Haworth Document Delivery Service: 1-800-HAWORTH. E-mail address: <docdelivery@haworthpress.com> Website: <http://www.Haworth Press.com> © 2007 by The Haworth Press, Inc. All rights reserved.]*

Diane E. Holland and Marcelline R. Harris are affiliated with Department of Nursing, Mayo Clinic College of Medicine, Rochester, MN.

[Haworth co-indexing entry note]: "Discharge Planning, Transitional Care, Coordination of Care, and Continuity of Care: Clarifying Concepts and Terms from the Hospital Perspective." Holland, Diane E. and Marcelline R. Harris. Co-published simultaneously in *Home Health Care Services Quarterly*® (The Haworth Press, Inc.) Vol. 26, No. 4, 2007, pp. 3-19; and: *Charting a Course for High Quality Care Transitions* (ed: Eric A. Coleman) The Haworth Press, Inc. 2007, pp. 3-19. Single or multiple copies of this article are available for a fee from The Haworth Document Delivery Service [1-800-HAWORTH, 9:00 a.m. - 5:00 p.m. (EST). E-mail address: docdelivery@haworthpress.com].

Available online at http://hhc.haworthpress.com
© 2007 by The Haworth Press, Inc. All rights reserved.
doi:10.1300/J027v26n04_02

KEYWORDS. Hospital discharge, discharge planning, transitional care, continuity of patient care, patient transfer, quality of healthcare, concept clarification, nursing models

INTRODUCTION

Patients and their families, providers, payers, and policy makers all share a longstanding concern about how to assure continuity of care. The relative prominence of this concern is noted in Institute of Medicine (IOM) documents focusing on the quality of health care and the "key challenge" of coordination of care across patient conditions, services, settings, and over time (IOM, 2001, 2003). Hospital discharge planning is widely recognized as a key process in achieving the outcome of continuity of care for persons leaving the hospital. The importance of hospital discharge planning in relation to continuity of care and the importance of continuity of care as a key indicator of quality of care is evident in, for example, the emphasis by various regulatory and accrediting agencies such as the Joint Commission (Joint Commission, 2006) and Centers for Medicare and Medicaid Services (CMS) (CFR, 2004; CMS, 2004). The emergence of electronic health records (EHRs) has brought another level of attention to this topic with national standards being proposed to address the fragmentation in the way information required for effective hospital discharge planning and continuity of care is captured, represented, and shared within the context of EHRs (HL7, 2007). Although an extensive body of literature that spans over 60 years has focused on hospital discharge planning and continuity of care, recent reviews of this literature note the limited scientific evidence to support causal associations and indicators of quality. In part, this is because the terms and concepts associated with hospital discharge planning, continuity of care, and quality are inconsistently defined and used. The inconsistent naming, definition and use of concepts is recognized as a barrier that inhibits the identification and adoption of best practices, and subsequent determinations of relevant aspects of the quality of care.

The purpose of this paper is to review the use of terms and definitions of key groups and literature reviews that have synthesized the content in this field and applied it to regulatory, accrediting, best practice recommendations, and quality of care determinations. We then (a) compare terms and definitions as they have been applied to inpatient, hospital based perspectives, and (b) propose a framework to facilitate consistent use of these concepts within the context of quality healthcare outcomes.

BACKGROUND

The literature on hospital discharge planning has developed over the last 60 years, beginning with descriptions of progressive patient care in hospitals and including the extension of hospital care into home care services (Abdellah & Levine, 1957). Hospital discharge planning became a more formal part of the national health policy with the enactment of Medicare and Medicaid in 1965. An increased national and interdisciplinary attention to discharge planning was evident in the 1970s, likely arising from a growing concern about the potential financial burden these two programs created for the federal government (Volland, 1988). By the 1980s, discharge planning had become a priority activity within many hospitals, motivated by the enactment of the Prospective Payment System (PPS) for Medicare and the amendment to the Social Security Act that required hospitals to have a discharge planning program as a condition of Medicare participation.

The literature on continuity of care appears to have emerged a bit later, perhaps in response to the increased focus on the implementation of hospital discharge planning. The first attempt to operationalize the concept of continuity of care in the United States can be traced to the early 1960s (Adair et al., 2003). Over time, the continuity of care literature has highlighted the evolution of hospital and medical care delivery beyond the hospital setting. Unfortunately, the meaning of continuity of care is more often presumed than defined in the literature. A recent review noted that at times it is impossible to infer the definition of the concept. "Where continuity is not explicitly defined, it's usually treated as a self evident concept of unquestionable good" (Reid, Haggerty, & McKendry, 2002, p. 2).

Since then related terms have been introduced in the literature. For example, transitional care emerged in the 1980s, linking home follow-up services provided after hospitalization with discharge planning during the patient's hospital stay (Brooten et al., 1986; Mary D. Naylor & McCauley, 1999; Phillips et al., 2004). Coordinated patient transitions from hospital to home are also referred to as 'seamless care' (Spehar et al., 2005). Fragmented care delivery and poor communication served as the impetus for the development of case management, another process that is believed to facilitate care coordination and care continuity (Chen, Brown, Archibald, Aliotta, & Fox, 2000). Overall, these terms are not well defined in the literature, and "are inextricably intermeshed and used interchangeably" (Harrison, Browen, Roberts, & Gafni, 1999, p. 315).

National organizations and federal agencies (e.g., Joint Commission, CMS, IOM) concerned with developing policy based on quality of care and other performance measures have focused a spotlight on hospital discharge planning and continuity of care. This has been motivated in part by a well recognized need to shape policy based on an understanding of the impacts of persons living longer with more chronic illnesses and the cost-effectiveness of different organizational models for delivering care. However, within the hospital provider community there is a widespread sense of "disconnect" among the resulting documents put forward by these groups. The following discussion presents a comparison of the definitions of concepts associated with hospital discharge planning, transitional care, coordination of care, and continuity of care across key regulatory, accrediting, and synthesis literature.

Applying a systematic approach to comparing concepts and terms is essential to understanding any subject field. It is important to note that philosophers of science have for centuries been debating which comes first, the concept (i.e., the abstract thought) or the term that names the concept (Rodgers & Knafl, 2000). Among the more widely used techniques for the analysis of concepts, there is agreement that the analysis requires one to examine the conditions and properties that are necessary to define a concept and sufficient to distinguish it from other concepts. Terms are then viewed as ways to name, and thus communicate about, concepts. While a structured concept analysis is beyond the scope of this article, reviewing definitions of terms is a way for us to determine in a somewhat objective fashion whether or not the same concept is being discussed across documents and to identify whether there is an implicit conceptual model in the literature that, if explicated, would facilitate ongoing efforts to develop common definition of concepts, terms, and relationships in the field.

METHODS

The approach we used to review definitions of discharge planning, transitional care, coordination of care, and continuity of care was to examine the agreement in synthesis or consensus documents regarding the concepts. Our review was limited to two types of documents that emphasized a hospital-focused perspective on policy or quality in this area: (1) white papers, regulations, and similar documents authored by national quality of care focused organizations and federal agencies that were published between January 2000 and December 2006, and (2) recent literature reviews. One criteria for including documents was the use of the keywords "discharge planning," "transitional care," "coordination of care" and "continuity of care." An additional refinement was a focus on the hospital to post-hospital transition. Therefore, we did not review documents that focused on intra-organizational continuity (e.g., within the hospital setting). We further excluded documents with a condition-specific focus (e.g., mental health, end of life care, congestive heart failure) because our interest here is in broadly applicable uses of the concepts and terms.

Two search strategies were used. First, search engines on web sites of relevant federal agencies and national quality of care-focused organizations were used to identify documents with the search terms. A determination of relevance was based on our own experience of the impact the organization or agency has on hospital practice. Second, a biomedical reference librarian conducted a search of MEDLINE, MEDLINE In-Process, and CINAHL databases to identify review articles captured by the search terms with truncations (truncation allows for all possible suffix variations of the root word) in the literature published in year 2000 to the present. Reports of meta-analyses were excluded, as our interest was in conceptualizations and definitions and not effects of different intervention strategies. For all documents identified by either strategy, we reviewed the reference lists to identify other organizations, agencies, or documents that we had not previously identified. The documents were then reviewed to identify terms and definitions associated with hospital discharge planning, transitional care, coordination of care, and continuity of care.

RESULTS

The final set of documents included nine from federal agencies and national quality of care focused organizations and six review articles. Table 1 identifies the web sites examined, the number of documents identified using the search terms, and the number of documents that met inclusion criteria for review. Of the 26 review articles identified, six met inclusion criteria for our review. Both authors reviewed the documents separately to identify terms and definitions. Differences were resolved by informal consensus. Table 2 summarizes the terms and definitions across documents retrieved from the web sites of federal agencies and quality of care focused organizations. Table 3 summarizes the terms and definitions across review articles, highlighting the question asked within the

TABLE 1. Documents Retrieved from Web Sites of Agencies and Organizations, Using Search Terms Discharge Planning, Transitional Care, Coordination of Care, or Continuity of Care

Web Site	Documents Identified (n)	Documents Meeting Inclusion Criteria (n)
Federal Agencies		
Centers for Medicare and Medicaid Strategies (http://www.cms.hhs.gov/)	54	3
Agency for Healthcare Research and Quality (http://www.ahrq.gov/)	1	0
− National Guideline Clearinghouse (http://www.guideline.gov/)	122	1
− National Quality Measures Clearinghouse (http://www.qualitymeasures.ahrq.gov/)	27	0
Canadian Health Services Research Foundation (http://www.chsrf.org/)	31	1
National Health Service Health Technology Assessment Programme (http://www.ncchta.org)	3	1
Quality of Care Focused Organizations		
Institute for Healthcare Improvement (http://www.ihi.org/ihi)	24	0
Institute of Medicine (http://www.iom.edu/)	2	0
Joint Commission (http://www.jointcommission.org/)	31	1
Leapfrog Group for Patient Safety (http://www.leapfroggroup.org/)	0	0
National Patient Safety Forum (http://www.npsf.org/)	2	0
National Quality Forum (http://www.qualityforum.org/)	13	1
EBM Reviews–Cochrane Database of Systematic Reviews	55	1

review that we believed lent insight into concept clarification and the number of articles included in the review. If no definition was provided, this was noted in the table.

Five of the six documents from federal agencies included the term 'discharge planning,' although none of these documents explicitly defined the term. Documents from the three national quality of care focused organizations had a mix of terms and definitions of 'continuity of care,' 'discharge planning,' and 'coordination of care.' Of the six review articles,

TABLE 2. Terms and Definitions Across Source Documents from Agencies and Organizations

Agency or Organization	Source Document	Defined Terms & Definitions
Federal Agencies		
CMS	42CFR 482.43 Condition of Participation: Discharge Planning (2004)	*Term: Discharge Planning* Not explicitly defined
	State Operations Manual (2004)	*Term: Discharge Planning* Not explicitly defined
(Health Care Financing Administration)	Best Practices in Coordinated Care (Chen et al., 2000)	*Term: Discharge Planning* Not explicitly defined
AHRQ–National Guideline Clearinghouse	Discharge Planning for the Older Adult (2003)	*Term: Discharge Planning* Not explicitly defined
Canadian Health Services Research Foundation	Defusing the Confusion: Concepts and measures of Continuity of Healthcare (Reid, Haggerty & McKendry, 2002)	*Term: Continuity of Care* There are two central elements that define continuity of care and form the base for understanding its three types. Continuity can only exist as an aspect of care that is experienced by an individual and that is received over time (p. 3)
National Health Service Health Technology Assessment Programme	A Systematic Review of Discharge Arrangements for Older People (Parker et al., 2002)	*Term: Discharge Planning* Not explicitly defined
National Quality of Care Focused Organizations		
Cochrane Collaboration	Discharge Planning from Hospital to Home (Parkes & Shepperd, 2006)	*Term: Discharge planning* The development of a discharge plan for the patient prior to leaving the hospital, with the aim of containing costs and improving patient outcomes (Plain Language Summary, ¶ 2)
The Joint Commission	Hospital Accreditation Standards (2006)	*Term(s): Discharge or Transfer* Not explicitly defined
National Quality Forum	National Voluntary Consensus Standards for Hospital Care: Additional Priority Areas (2006)	*Term: Coordination of Care* Not explicitly defined

TABLE 3. Terms and Definitions Across Review Articles

Review Article	Review Question(s) Most Relevant to Concept Clarification	Keywords Used (alone or in combination)	# Articles Reviewed	Defined Terms and Definitions
(Bull, 2000)	• What is known about discharge planning for older people?	Patient discharge, elderly or aged, research or study	288	*Term: Discharge Planning* An interdisciplinary process that assesses the need for follow-up care and arranges for that care, whether self-care, care provided by family members, care from health professionals or a combination of these options (p. 70).
(Donaldson, 2001)	• Might the study findings have provided useful direction for further research and policy making if the study design and analysis had drawn on the agency model of continuity?	Continuity of patient care, economics, statistics & numerical data, clinical trial, controlled clinical trial, cross-sectional studies, multivariate analysis	49	*Term: Continuity of Care* An intervening variable that may affect agency by decreasing information asymmetry and increasing goal alignment (p. 261)
Helleso & Lorensen (2005)	• How is inter-organizational continuity of care described and defined? • What structural components are associated with continuity of care?	Continuity of care, electronic patient record	41	*Term: Inter-organizational continuity of care* The formal and informal communication, coordination, and structure and unstructured information exchange at an individual and organizational level (p. 819)
(Naylor, 2002)	• What is known about the effectiveness of existing processes of care and innovative interventions designed to address the needs of elders and their caregivers who are making transitions across settings or from one level of care to another?	Transitional care, Discharge planning, Care coordination, Case management, Continuity of care, Referrals, Post-discharge follow-up, Patient assessment, Patient needs, Interventions, Evaluation	94	*Term: Transitional Care* A term that encompasses a range of services and environments designed to promote the safe and timely transfer of patients from one level of care to another (p. 128)

Source	Questions	Keywords		Term
(Sparbel and Anderson, 2000)	• How has continuity of care been defined in the nursing literature? • What factors, variables, and concepts are significant to continuity of care?	Continuity of care, Patient discharge		*Term: Continuity of Care* A multidimensional term used to describe a variety of relationships between patients and the delivery of health care (p. 128)
			38	*Term: Continuity of Care* A series of connected patient-care events both within a health care institution and among multiple settings (p.17)
(van Servellen et al., 2006)	• Which type(s) of continuity of care was/were addressed?	Continuity of patient care, Quality of care	32	*Term: Continuity of Care* Coherent patient care over time and setting (p. 185)

11

'continuity of care' was found more often that 'discharge planning,' perhaps reflecting the timeframe we imposed for the literature review.

Hospital Discharge Planning

Hospital discharge planning definitions, although few in number, appear to indicate that it is a process that is bounded by the length of inpatient stays (Bull, 2000; Parkes & Shepperd, 2004).

Transitional Care

Only one definition of transitional care was found in our review documents. Transitional care, like discharge planning, was defined as a process of care; however, the definition was not specific regarding events that denote the start and end of transitional care (Naylor, 2002). In fact, transitional care is typically described with respect to the support services, follow-up activities, and other interventions that span pre-hospital discharge to post-hospital settings (Coleman, 2003; Coleman & Boult, 2003; M. D. Naylor et al., 2004). This is in contrast to discharge planning, which is bounded by a hospital admission and discharge event.

Coordination of Care

Coordination of care was also considered a concept generally understood by healthcare providers (NQF, 2006) with no explicit definition found in any of the documents. Discussions of coordination of care focus on the integration or sequencing of activities of care (Reid et al., 2002). The emphasis is on linking planning and management activities across different providers, recording that information into a summative document (e.g., a care plan), and also linking those planning and management efforts and interventions into a care delivery system (e.g., organizational work units and the people who work in organizational systems). The goal appears to be a coherent scheme of management. Viewed this way coordination of care can be seen as an attribute of both discharge planning and transitional care; but coordination of care is not an intervention in and of itself. Furthermore, coordination of care done well appears to influence management continuity outcomes.

Continuity of Care

Five definitions of continuity of care were found. The focus of continuity of care definitions were for the most part not process oriented, but instead focused on the outcomes and the relatedness and interactions among care delivery mechanisms and providers, patients, and family (Haggerty et al., 2003; Naylor, 2002; Sparbel & Anderson, 2000). Attributes of continuity of care that seem to differentiate this concept from other related concepts include a focus on the patient and an element of temporality (Reid et al., 2002; van Servellen, Fongwa, & D'Errico, 2006). Continuity is not considered a characteristic of providers or organizations (Reid et al., 2002).

Three types of continuity were mentioned repeatedly: informational, relational or interpersonal, and management continuity. Informational continuity exists when information on prior events experienced by patients is available and used to provide care appropriate to the patient's current circumstances (Haggerty et al., 2003; van Servellen et al., 2006). Relational or interpersonal continuity refers to an ongoing therapeutic relationship between provider and patient characterized by personal trust and responsibility that provides a link to future care (Haggerty et al., 2003). Management continuity discussions in the literature typically referred to use of protocols and guidelines to assure care or treatment from more than one provider is connected, orderly, coherent, complementary, and timely (Haggerty et al., 2003; van Servellen et al., 2006).

Informational continuity has been the historical focus of discharge planning. Informational continuity is considered necessary for continuity over time (chronologic), although several authors discussing informational continuity remarked that much of the knowledge required to bridge the provision of services across providers and settings is highly tacit and not made explicit in documentation. Not surprisingly, informational continuity is the focus of the EHR community. Recently, a standard entitled the "Continuity of Care Document" (CCD) passed balloting by HL7, one of the standards development organization used by federal agencies to develop and implement new healthcare information technology systems. The CCD standard represents an intensive collaboration effort to define a continuity of care record as a minimum dataset "consisting of the most relevant and timely facts about a patient's condition" a healthcare provider needs to make decisions (Ferranti, Musser, Kawamoto, & Hammond, 2006; HL7, 2007). A set of technical specifications were then applied to this data set to address the requirements of providers within and across disciplines to easily access and update information as patients transition across providers and settings.

Relational or interpersonal continuity is emphasized in the literature on patient-doctor relationships and may reflect the ongoing relationship between physician and patient that are typically not setting bound; although it is noted that the effect of physician hospitalists has an unknown effect on this type of continuity (Adair et al., 2003; Donaldson, Yordy, Lohr, & Vanselow, 1996; Jee, 2006; Wenger & Young, 2004). Disciplines such as nursing and social work have historically focused efforts on discharge planning interventions in the setting within which they are employed. While there is a rich literature within each of those disciplines describing relational continuity, it tends to be bounded by the setting with the notable exceptions of Brooten and Naylor's work with transitional care (Naylor et al., 2004).

Van Servellen (2006) posits that management continuity, focusing on the procedural aspects of assuring continuity, is required for both informational and relational continuity. Haggerty (2003) referred to these as different 'types' and 'attributes' of continuity of care. At times a discussion of continuity served as the definition for continuity of care (van Servellen et al., 2006).

The discussion above suggests that there is a common conceptual model underlying the concepts of discharge planning, transitional care, coordination of care, and continuity of care. Below, we discuss that model, emphasizing the use of these concepts within the context of healthcare quality.

CONCEPTUAL MODEL

For more than four decades Donabedian's conceptualization of structure, process, and outcome indicators has influenced the study of healthcare quality in general (Donabedian, 1966) and hospital discharge planning specifically (Donabedian & Rosenfeld, 1964). A large body of literature on the measurement of indicators of structure, process, outcome, and characteristics of individuals within care delivery systems (i.e., provider, patient and family) has resulted. More recent efforts in conceptualizations of quality have focused on the challenge of trying to classify and develop taxonomies that assist in sorting and classifying indicators of concepts and processes and specifying relationships between and among component parts. For example, Holzemer and Reilly (1995) built on Donebedian's structure, process, and outcome conceptualization and additionally incorporate the variability often introduced by patients, providers, and organizations. Mitchell, Ferketich and Jennings (1998) proposed a model which incorporates concepts from the work of both Donebedian and Holzemer and Reilly, but graphically illustrates the direct and indirect interactions that must be considered when trying to estimate quality outcomes. This is consistent with the model proposed by Donaldson (2001) that focused specifically on a conceptualization of continuity of care. McBryde-Foster and Allen (2005) focused on the continuum of care as a summative entity, defining continuum of care as a "series of initiating, continuing and concluding care events," noting that "over time, the patient progresses between environments of care through events called transition points" (p. 630).

Jointly, these conceptualizations suggest a "meta-structure' into which concepts such as discharge planning, transitional care, coordination of care and continuity of care can be sorted and placed. Figure 1 illustrates a conceptual model that accommodates the definitions discussed above. Continuity of care is an outcome in and of itself, but can also serve as an intervening variable in other, typically more distant in time, quality of care outcomes such as readmission, satisfaction, self-care, etc. Additionally, continuity of care can be sub-typed as informational continuity, relational continuity, and management continuity. Discharge planning is a process (or set of interventions) that is bounded by admission and discharge to specific settings of care (in this case hospital), while transitional care is a process that spans settings of care (in this case pre-hospital discharge to post hospital settings) with no events that consistently signal start and stop points. Coordination of care is an attribute of both discharge planning and

FIGURE 1. Conceptual Framework for Positioning Hospital Discharge Planning within the Context of Quality Health Outcomes*

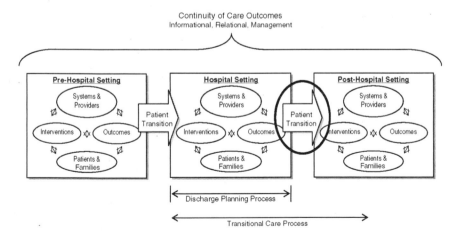

* Adapted from Mitchell PH, Ferketich S & Jennings B. (1998). Quality Health Outcomes Model. *Image, 30*(1), 43-46 and McBryde-Foster, M. & Allen, T. (2005). The continuum of care: A concept development study. *Journal of Advanced Nursing, 50*(6), 624-632.

transitional care and is not useful to be considered an intervention in and of itself. The figure specifically calls out discharge planning and transitional care in order to emphasize the time and setting dimensions of these interventions.

TAKE HOME POINTS

1. Consensus on terms and definitions is foundational to developing indicators of evidence based processes, interventions and quality healthcare outcomes.
2. The concepts of hospital discharge planning, transitional care, coordination of care, and continuity of care are interrelated.
3. We will continue to struggle with scientific progress and translating that science into practice and policy until we come to agreement on the use of terms and definitions for hospital discharge planning and related concepts.

CONCLUSION

The concepts of discharge planning, transitional care, coordination of care, and continuity of care are clearly important in the current health care policy and in both hospital and home healthcare practice environments. More than semantic quibbling, it is critical that we sort through the current use of terms and definitions and move towards consensus on what we mean with the words we use. The definitions and conceptual model proposed above can clarify future discussions of these key concepts in relationship to indicators of quality healthcare processes and outcomes.

This paper does not represent a complete systematic review. Given our rather narrow inclusion criteria, and our attempt to review documents that apply to broad types of patients leaving the hospital, we did not include information in the condition-specific and the discipline specific literature (e.g., family practice community perspective of continuity of care). Additionally, we did not review the literature that focuses on measurement and indicators of each of the concepts discussed in this paper. The conceptualization described above is only an abstraction from current "synthesis documents" and requires evaluation using research methodologies. To that end, the authors invite discussion and further development of this framework for its value in guiding research, practice, and policy for discharge planning, transitional care, coordination of care, and continuity of care.

REFERENCES

Abdellah, F. G., & Levine, E. (1957). Polling patients and personnel–part 4: What hospitals have done to improve patient care. *Hospitals, Journal of the American Hospital Association, 31*, 43-44.

Adair, C. E., McDougall, G. M., Beckie, A., Joyce, A., Mitton, C., Wild, C. T. et al. (2003). History and measurement of continuity of care in mental health services and evidence of its role in outcomes. *Psychiatric Services, 54*(10), 1351-1356. doi:10.1176/appi.ps.54.10.1351

Brooten, D., Kumar, S., Brown, L. P., Butts, P., Finkler, S. A., Bakewell-Sachs, S. et al. (1986). A randomized clinical trial of early hospital discharge and home follow-up of very-low-birth-weight infants. *New England Journal of Medicine, 315*(15), 934-939.

Bull, M. J. (2000). Discharge planning for older people: A review of current research. *British Journal of Community Nursing, 5*(2), 70-74.

CFR. (2004). Code of Federal Regulations, Title 42: Public Health (69 FR 49268), *Standards for Hospital Discharge Planning: Social Security Act Section 1861, Subsection (ee)*.

Chen, A., Brown, R., Archibald, N., Aliotta, S., & Fox, P. D. (2000). *Best practices in coordinated care* (No. HCFA 500-95-0048 (04)). Baltimore, MD: Health Care Financing Administration.

CMS. (2004). *State Operations Manual: Appendix A-Survey protocol, regulations and Interpretive guidelines for hospitals*. Retrieved Nov. 01, 2006, from http://www.cms.hhs.gov/manuals/downloads/som107ap_a_hospitals.pdf.

Coleman, E. A. (2003). Falling through the cracks: Challenges and opportunities for improving transitional care for persons with continuous complex care needs. *Journal of the American Geriatrics Society, 51*(4), 549-555. doi:10.1046/j.1532-5415.2003.51185.x

Coleman, E. A., & Boult, C. (2003). Improving the quality of transitional care for persons with complex care needs: Position statement of The American Geriatrics Society Health Care Systems Committee. *Journal of the American Geriatrics Society, 51*, 556-557. doi:10.1046/j.1532-5415.2003.51186.x

Donabedian, A. (1966). Evaluating the quality of medical care. *Milbank Memorial Fund Quarterly, 44*(part 2), 166-206. doi:10.2307/3348969

Donabedian, A., & Rosenfeld, L. S. (1964). Follow-up study of chronically ill patients discharged from hospital. *Journal of Chronic Diseases, 17*(9), 847-862. doi:10.1016/0021-9681(64)90013-X

Donaldson, M. S. (2001). Continuity of care: A reconceptualization. *Medical Care Research and Review, 58*(3), 255-290.

Donaldson, M. S., Yordy, K. D., Lohr, K. N., & Vanselow, N. A. (1996). *Primary care: America's health in a new era*: The National Academies Press.

Ferranti, J. M., Musser, R. C., Kawamoto, K., & Hammond, W. E. (2006). The clinical document architecture and the continuity of care record: A critical analysis. *Journal of the American Informatics Association, 13,* 245-252. doi:10.1197/jamia.M1963

Haggerty, J. L., Reid, R. J., Freeman, G. K., Starfield, B. H., Adair, C. E., & McKendry, R. (2003). Continuity of care: A multidisciplinary review. *British Medical Journal, 327,* 1219-1221. doi:10.1136/bmj.327.7425.1219

Harrison, M. B., Browen, B. G., Roberts, J., & Gafni, A. (1999). Understanding continuity of care and how to bridge the intersectoral gaps: A planning and evaluation framework. *National Academies of Practice Forum: Issues in Interdisciplinary Care, 1*(4), 315-326.

HL7. (2007). *HL7 Continuity of Care Document, a healthcare IT interoperability standard, is approved by balloting process and endorsed by healthcare IT standards panel.* Retrieved February 16, 2007, from http://www.hl7.org/press/PressReleases RSS.cfm.

Holzemer, W. L., & Reilly, C. A. (1995). Variables, variability, and variations research: Implications for medical informatics. *Journal of the American Medical Informatics Association, 2*(3), 183-190.

IOM. (2001). *Crossing the quality chasm.* Washington, DC: National Academies Press.

IOM (Ed.). (2003). *Priority areas for national action: Transforming health care quality.* Washington, DC: National Academy Press.

Jee, S. H. (2006). Indices for continuity of care: A systematic review of the literature. *Medical Care Research and Review, 63*(2), 158-188. doi:10.1177/1077558705285294

McBryde-Foster, M., & Allen, T. (2005). The continuum of care: A concept development study. *Journal of Advanced Nursing, 50*(6), 624-632. doi:10.1111/j.1365-2648. 2005.03447.x

Mitchell, P. A., Ferketich, S., & Jennings, B. M. (1998). Quality health outcomes model. *Image–the Journal of Nursing Scholarship, 30*(1), 43-46.

Naylor, M. D. (2002). Transitional care of older adults. In P. Archbold & B. Stewart (Eds.), *Annual Review of Nursing Research* (Vol. 20, pp. 127-147). New York: Springer.

Naylor, M. D., & McCauley, K. M. (1999). The effects of a discharge planning and home follow-up intervention on elders hospitalized with common medical and surgical cardiac conditions. *Journal of Cardiovascular Nursing, 14*(1), 44-54.

Naylor, M. D., Brooten, D. A., Campbell, R. L., Maislin, G., McCauley, K. M., Schwartz, J. S. et al. (2004). Transitional care of older adults hospitalized with heart failure: A randomized, controlled trial. *Journal of the American Geriatrics Society, 52*(5), 675-684. doi:10.1111/j.1532-5415.2004.52202.x

NQF. (2006). *National voluntary consensus standards for hospital care: Additional priority areas–2005-2006.* Washington, DC: National Quality Forum.

Parker, S. G., Peet, S. M., McPherson, A., Cannaby, A. M., Abrams, K., Baker, R. et al. (2002). A systematic review of discharge arrangements for older people. *Health Technology Assessment, 6*(4), 1-183.

Parkes, J., & Shepperd, S. (2004). Discharge planning from hospital to home. *Cochrane Database of Systematic Reviews*(2).

Phillips, C. O., Wright, S. M., Kern, D. E., Singa, R. M., Shepperd, S., & Rubin, H. R. (2004). Comprehensive discharge planning with postdischarge support for older patients with congestive heart failure. *Journal of the American Medical Association, 291*(11), 1358-1367. doi:10.1001/jama.291.11.1358

Reid, R., Haggerty, J., & McKendry, R. (2002). *Defusing the confusion: Concepts and measures of continuity of healthcare.* Ottawa, Ontario: Canadian Health Services Research Foundation.

Rodgers, B. L., & Knafl, K. A. (Eds.). (2000). *Concept development in nursing: Foundations, techniques, and applications* (2nd ed.). Philadelphia, PA: W.B. Saunders Company.

Sparbel, K. J. H., & Anderson, M. A. (2000). Integrated literature review of continuity of care: Part 1, conceptual issues. *Journal of Nursing Scholarship, 32*(1), 17-24. doi:10.1111/j.1547-5069.2000.00017.x

Spehar, A. M., Campbell, R. R., Cherrie, C., Palacios, P., Scott, D., Baker, J. L. et al. (2005). *Seamless care: Safe patient transitions from hospital to home.* Retrieved Nov. 10, 2006, from http://www.ahrq.gov/downloads/pub/advances/vol1/Spehar.pdf.

van Servellen, G., Fongwa, M., & D'Errico, E. M. (2006). Continuity of care and quality care outcomes for people experiencing chronic conditions: A literature review. *Nursing and Health Sciences, 8*, 185-195. doi:10.1111/j.1442-2018.2006.00278.x

Volland, P. J. (Ed.). (1988). *Discharge planning: An interdisciplinary approach to continuity of care.* Owings Mills, MD: National Health Publishing.

Wenger, N. S., & Young, R. (2004). *Quality indicators of continuity and coordination of care for vulnerable elder persons.* Santa Monica, CA: Rand Health.

doi:10.1300/J027v26n04_02

Development and Testing of an Analytic Model to Identify Home Healthcare Patients at Risk for a Hospitalization Within the First 60 Days of Care

Robert J. Rosati, PhD
Liping Huang, MA

SUMMARY. Preventing hospitalization is one of the major objectives of home health care. Accomplishing this goal is being able to identify patients at risk for hospitalization and intervening appropriately. The current study explored which factors place patients at risk at the start of care and are predictive over the first 60 days of care. Outcomes Assessment Information Set (OASIS), plan of care, medications and medical record information from an urban home health agency were used to build and validate a

Robert J. Rosati is Director of Outcomes Analysis and Research at the Center for Home Care Policy and Research, Visiting Nurse Service of New York. Liping Huang is Lead Biostatistics Analyst at Hoffmann-La Roche Ltd., and was previously a Senior Statistical Analyst at the Center for Home Care Policy and Research, Visiting Nurse Service of New York.

Address correspondence to: Robert J. Rosati, PhD, Center for Home Care Policy and Research, Visiting Nurse Service of New York, 1250 Broadway, 20th Floor, New York, NY 10001 (E-mail: Robert.Rosati@vnsny.org)

The authors would like to thank Sally Sobolewski, RN, and James Budis, RN, for their clinical input related to the risk model and the time spent conducting the blinded record reviews.

[Haworth co-indexing entry note]: "Development and Testing of an Analytic Model to Identify Home Healthcare Patients at Risk for a Hospitalization Within the First 60 Days of Care." Rosati, Robert J., and Liping Huang. Co-published simultaneously in *Home Health Care Services Quarterly*® (The Haworth Press, Inc.) Vol. 26, No. 4, 2007, pp. 21-36; and: *Charting a Course for High Quality Care Transitions* (ed: Eric A. Coleman) The Haworth Press, Inc. 2007, pp. 21-36. Single or multiple copies of this article are available for a fee from The Haworth Document Delivery Service [1-800-HAWORTH, 9:00 a.m. - 5:00 p.m. (EST). E-mail address: docdelivery@haworthpress.com].

predictive hospitalization model. The model was developed and tested using a large set of patients (n = 46,366). Patients were classified into seven risk groups from very low to very high. Results revealed that a combination of demographic, financial, clinical and health status factors could accurately predict patients' likelihood for hospitalization and the model agreed with clinical judgments. Examples of how the risk model could be used in practice are provided. doi:10.1300/J027v26n04_03 *[Article copies available for a fee from The Haworth Document Delivery Service: 1-800-HAWORTH. E-mail address: <docdelivery@haworthpress.com> Website: <http://www.HaworthPress.com> © 2007 by The Haworth Press, Inc. All rights reserved.]*

KEYWORDS. Homecare, OASIS, hospitalization, outcome measurement, quality improvement

INTRODUCTION

Home health care is in the forefront of providing post acute care services to an aging and typically acutely ill patient population. Many of these patients are at high risk of being hospitalized for the first time (i.e., community referral) or rehospitalized (i.e., hospital referral). There is significant economic cost related to hospitalization, which can be measured in terms of the impact on patients, families, and society. The ability to intervene early with patients at high risk for hospitalization could have potential benefits by improving the quality of care, utilizing services appropriately and reducing the cost of delivery care. The challenge is being able to identify these patients using information readily available to home health agencies when they enter into care.

Background and Existing Literature

In 2002 the Centers for Medicare and Medicaid Service (CMS) implemented outcome-based quality improvement (OBQI) indicators for home health care agencies to improvement the measurement of patient outcomes and for monitoring services provided by home health care agencies (Centers for Medicare and Medicaid Services, 2002). Part of OBQI is the inclusion of an indicator of acute care hospitalization (Shaughnessy et al., 2002). Since OBQI measures became publicly reported by CMS in 2004 on the Home Health Compare web site (www.medicare.gov), the national rate of acute care hospitalization for home health care Medicare patients has remained relatively stable. For example when comparing two reports from 2004 and 2006 there was little change in hospitalization rates: January to December 2004 was 28.0% and April 2005 to March 2006 was 28.4% (Centers for Medicare and Medicaid Services, 2006). Based on these statistics it can be assumed that at least half of all of home health care agencies have risk adjusted acute care hospitalization rates of higher than 28%. Therefore, reducing home health care hospitalization rates should be an important objective for both policy makers and health care providers. Further, this measure of agency performance is likely to become a major factor in future efforts by CMS to pay for performance (Humphrey, 2005).

Although hospitalization may be an unavoidable consequence due to declining health or a traumatic incident, it is clear from the variation in agency risk-adjusted rates across the country that there is an opportunity to prevent unnecessary acute care hospitalizations. The ability to predict the risk of hospitalization can help clinicians identify appropriate interventions for patients and potentially prevent hospitalizations. Risk assessment could enhance care planning to differentiate between those who may need more intense services, like placing remote monitors in the home and those patients who may need less intense service (i.e., fewer certified visits). Currently, there is limited research on using home health care specific data like the OASIS and other patient information (e.g., plan of care, medications, vital signs) in predicting the risk of hospitalization, especially factors related to earlier onset of hospitalization. A study by Rosati, Huang, Navaie-Waliser and Feldman (2003) did show that the OASIS, clinical and demographic data could be used to identify home health care patients who have repeated hospitalizations. However, beyond home health care there is a substantial literature evaluating other types of information in predicting hospitalization, mostly related to discharges from a hospital setting. For example, Coleman et al., (1998) found that administrative data could identify patients at risk for hospitalization and functional declines. Administrative data was also found to be useful in classify patients at risk for a complicated transition from the hospital to post hospital care (Coleman, Min, Chomiak & Kramer, 2004). Other research has focused on validating a self-administered risk assessment tool, called the Pra, which could be used with any older individual (age > 60 or 65), living in the community, to predict hospitalization risk (e.g., Boult, Boult, Pirie & Pacala, 1994; Wagner et al., 2006).

Potential Risk Factors

The existing literature suggests that possible predictors of the risk of hospitalization include demographic characteristics, type of insurance, severity of illness, readiness for hospital discharge, the quality and quantity of home health care services provided, the availability of an informal caregiver, suitability of the home environment and degree of social isolation. Other factors that have been linked to hospitalization include the complexity of treatment associated with specific health conditions (such as congestive heart failure, type of wound, hypertension, acquired immunodeficiency syndrome, and diabetes) and the associated patient compliance with medication regimens (Anderson, Helms, Hanson & DeVilder, 1999; Gautam, Macduff, Brown & Squair, 1996; Kliebsch, Siebert & Brenner, 2000; Rosati et al., 2003; Schwarz, 2000).

Current Study

The purposes of the current study was to identify risk factors that are associated with events of acute care hospitalization within 60 days of admission to home health care using data that is readily available at start of care, build a model to predict risk, test the validity of the model to accurately predict hospitalization and attempt to use the risk model to assist clinicians in their care planning.

METHODS

Study Design and Data

The study is based on retrospective data from a large urban home healthcare agency. Patients who were admitted to an adult acute care program during September 2004 through April 2005, and an Outcomes Assessment Information Set (OASIS) collected at start of care (n = 46,366).[1] In addition to the OASIS assessment, supplemental information was gathered on patient demographics, medications, social supports and clinical status. These data came from the plan of care (CMS-485) and the agency's electronic medical record. Furthermore, if a patient was served by the agency in the prior 6 months of the admission, the administrative information from the previous admission was included as well (n = 10,822, 23.3%). The complete data set included the following domains: patient demographics characteristics (e.g., age, gender, race, insurance carrier, and education level), social supports (e.g., living arrangement, caregiver), previous case history (e.g., had hospitalization, emergent care, or nursing home stay prior admission), clinical and mental status (e.g., diagnosis and its severity at admission, comborbidities, pain management, medication regimen, temperature, blood pressure, pulse, and cognitive impairment), functional status specific to activity of daily living such as bathing, transferring, and instrumental activities of daily such as preparing light means, self-transporting, doing laundry, and medication utilization such as the number of medications taken at start of care, and if there was an existing medication reaction. Data from the plan of care included physician authorized professional and paraprofessional services.

Statistical Analysis

Statistical analyses were performed using SAS statistical software. The analyses for building the hospitalization model were conducted using several steps. First, descriptive analyses for the independent variables were derived for all domains of data. Second, chi-square tests (or Fisher exact test as appropriate) and t-test were used to assess for significance for relationships between patients who had hospitalization within 60 days of admission versus who were not have hospitalization. Third, the complete data set was randomly split into two sets: one for the modeling and the other for validation purposes. Based on the initial examination of the data, a logistic regression model with stepwise variable selection was estimated to identify risk factors related to the likelihood of hospitalization within the 60 days of home care admission. The mathematic equation related to the logistic regression model was formulated as the

$$\log\left(\frac{\pi}{1-\pi}\right) = \alpha + \beta X$$

following: π denotes the probability of admitted to hospitals within 60 days of start of care, X denotes a matrix of covariates, and α is the intercept of the liner regression model. After the model was defined, the statistically significant risk factors were examined by a team of clinical experts at the agency for conceptual considerations, and the model was modified based on clinical input. The final stage of the analysis was validating the model. The calibration and ability of the model to discriminate between patients with and without hospitalization were assessed using the Hosmer-Lemeshow statistic and C-indices, respectively. Furthermore, by examining the distribution of the predicted probabilities as well as the sensitivity and specificity from modeling results, appropriate cutoff points were determined to categorize patients into seven different risk groups, ranging from very low risk to very high risk. After developing the risk-adjusted model using the modeling data set, the model was applied to the validation data set and patients were divided into risk groups. A comparison was then made of the actual hospitalization rates between the modeling and validation data sets, at each risk level, to evaluate the predictability, accuracy and stability of the model. To establish whether the model concurred with clinical judgments about patient risk for a hospitalization, the clinical experts conducted 25 blinded record reviews. Two clinicians were asked to judge the level of risk for a hospitalization using the same seven-point scale established for classifying patients by the model (very low, low, low moderate, moderate, moderate high, high, very high). Clinical judgments were restricted to only information available at the start of care. Kappa statistics were computed to assess the level of agreement between the two clinicians and the risk score calculated by the model.

RESULTS

Table 1 shows the descriptive analyses and bivariate comparisons for the entire sample of patients (n = 46,366). As can be seen in Table 1, the hospitalized and non-hospitalized groups are significantly different on almost every domain (e.g., demographics, insurance, general health status, physician authorized visits). In general the hospitalized group was slightly older, more likely to be dually eligible (Medicare and Medicaid), living alone, had history of hospitalization or emergent care, poorer health status and more certified visits at start of care. The overall hospitalization rate within 60 days of admission was 19.9% (n = 9,229). Most patients (50.1%) were hospitalized within 14 days, with the percentage decreasing over the 60 days: 15-30 days 28.0%, 31-45 days 13.7% and 46-60 days 8.2%.

Table 2 includes the final model used to predict hospitalization based on the random half of the sample selected for model development (n = 23,079). The logistic model was statistically significant (Likelihood Ratio = 1986.7, df = 51, p < .0001) and had a c-statistic = 0.71. The c-statistic is a measure of model discrimination and is 1.0 when a model perfectly predicts an outcome. When a model cannot discriminate (i.e., cases have randomly predicted outcomes) the c-statistic is 0.5. Values of less than 0.5 indicate improper coding of predicted and actual outcomes. The

TABLE 1. Descriptive Statistics

	No Event of Hospitalization (N = 36,984)	Had an Event of Hospitalization within First 60 Days (N = 9,175)	Probability
Age			
Age (mean)	70.31	71.01	0.0002
Age 18-54 (%)	17.5%	15.9%	0.0001
Age 55-64 (%)	14.8%	14.5%	0.5140
Age 65-74 (%)	19.9%	21.2%	0.0046
Age 75-84 (%)	28.0%	27.8%	0.6681
Age ≥ 85 (%)	19.8%	20.6%	0.0697
Gender			
Female (%)	64.3%	60.8%	<.0001
Race			
White (%)	50.7%	45.9%	<.0001
Hispanic (%)	20.5%	23.4%	<.0001
Payer			
Medicare FFS (%)	39.3%	40.1%	0.2007
Medicaid FFS (%)	8.8%	10.9%	<.0001
Dually Eligible (%)	19.5%	24.2%	<.0001
Medicare HMO (%)	9.0%	8.0%	0.004
Medicaid HMO (%)	5.4%	4.6%	0.0018
Private Insurance HMO (%)	15.1%	10.5%	<.0001
Other (%)	1.0%	0.3%	<.0001
No Charge (%)	1.8%	1.4%	0.0097
Education			
Higher than Graduate (%)	4.9%	4.2%	0.0024
Living Arrangement			
Alone (%)	33.9%	31.7%	0.0001
Previous Case History			
Had Previous Cases Prior 6 Months (%)	21.1%	32.2%	<.0001
# of Hospitalization Prior 6 Months	0.7741	0.9728	<.0001
Had Hospitalization Prior 30 Days (%)	72.5%	78.8%	<.0001
General Health Status			
Poor Prognosis (%)	9.0%	17.1%	<.0001
Rehab Guarded (%)	21.8%	33.2%	<.0001
Life Expectancy ≤ 6 Months (%)	2.0%	4.2%	<.0001

TABLE 1 (continued)

	No Event of Hospitalization (N = 36,984)	Had an Event of Hospitalization within First 60 Days (N = 9,175)	Probability
Certified Visits By Physicians			
Nursing (mean)	27.49	31.66	<.0001
HHA (mean)	17.22	22.32	<.0001
Social Work (mean)	1.09	1.62	<.0001

TABLE 2. Model for Predicting Hospitalization within the First 60 Days of Admission

					Odds Ratio		
Parameter	Estimate	Standard Error	Wald Chi-Square	Probability	Odds Ratio	Lower 95% CI	Upper 95% CI
Intercept	−2.446	0.175	195.102	<.0001			
Demographics							
Assessment completed by nurse	0.582	0.177	10.764	0.001	1.789	1.264	2.532
Female	−0.135	0.037	13.464	0.000	0.874	0.813	0.939
Caregiver others (ref: no caregiver)	0.104	0.049	4.405	0.036	1.109	1.007	1.222
Insurance (Ref: Medicaid FFS)							
Private HMO	−0.230	0.057	16.010	<.0001	0.795	0.710	0.890
Other Payer	−0.673	0.296	5.177	0.023	0.510	0.286	0.911
No Charge	−0.330	0.162	4.135	0.042	0.719	0.523	0.988
Previous Cases History							
Had case(s) opened prior 6 months	0.175	0.045	15.338	<.0001	1.192	1.092	1.301
Number of hospitalization prior 6 months	0.134	0.045	8.795	0.003	1.143	1.047	1.249
Number of emergent care prior 6 months	0.214	0.047	20.398	<.0001	1.238	1.129	1.359
Had rehab history prior 6 months	−0.233	0.054	18.297	<.0001	0.792	0.712	0.882
Certified Service Utilization at Admission Certified Nursing Visit for 60 Days (Ref: No Visits Needed)							
1-7(6%)	−0.342	0.220	2.427	0.119	0.710	0.462	1.092

TABLE 2 (continued)

Parameter	Estimate	Standard Error	Wald Chi-Square	Probability	Odds Ratio	Lower 95% CI	Upper 95% CI
8-18 (11.4%)	−0.155	0.214	0.523	0.470	0.857	0.564	1.303
19-26 (7.71%)	0.050	0.216	0.054	0.817	1.051	0.689	1.605
27 (30.51%)	0.013	0.209	0.004	0.949	1.013	0.673	1.527
28-39 (30.13%)	0.160	0.210	0.582	0.446	1.174	0.778	1.771
40-63 (6.69%)	0.427	0.218	3.846	0.050	1.533	1.000	2.350
>63 (2.76%)	0.258	0.231	1.250	0.264	1.295	0.823	2.037
Certified HHA Visit for 60 Days (Ref: No Visits Needed)							
1-45 (27.87%)	0.134	0.042	10.031	0.002	1.143	1.052	1.242
>45 (11.57%)	0.158	0.055	8.428	0.004	1.171	1.053	1.303
Certified Social Work Visits (Ref: No Visits Needed)							
1-5 (5.2%)	0.177	0.075	5.572	0.018	1.193	1.030	1.382
6-8 (5.4%)	0.241	0.072	11.276	0.001	1.272	1.105	1.464
>8 (4.5%)	0.244	0.078	9.831	0.002	1.276	1.096	1.486
Information at admission							
No inpatient discharge	−0.265	0.059	20.118	<.0001	0.767	0.683	0.861
Rehab guarded	0.215	0.040	28.416	<.0001	1.239	1.145	1.341
Diagnoses							
4 or more illness	0.076	0.037	4.211	0.040	1.079	1.003	1.161
CHF	0.279	0.065	18.585	<.0001	1.322	1.164	1.500
Ischemic heart disease	0.201	0.077	6.880	0.009	1.222	1.052	1.420
HIV	0.347	0.123	7.948	0.005	1.414	1.111	1.799
Cancer	0.698	0.055	163.520	<.0001	2.010	1.806	2.236
Injury or Poisoning	−0.255	0.078	10.734	0.001	0.775	0.666	0.903
Diabetes with complication of wound	0.259	0.055	21.879	<.0001	1.296	1.163	1.445
Renal Failure (Ref: no renal failure)	0.553	0.113	23.914	<.0001	1.738	1.393	2.170
Renal Failure with dialysis (Ref: no renal failure)	0.649	0.093	48.520	<.0001	1.913	1.594	2.297
Combination of comorbidity and severity	0.012	0.004	8.731	0.003	1.012	1.004	1.020
Clinical Status							
Unhealed pressure ulcer	0.345	0.124	7.795	0.005	1.413	1.108	1.800

TABLE 2 (continued)

Parameter	Estimate	Standard Error	Wald Chi-Square	Probability	Odds Ratio		
					Odds Ratio	Lower 95% CI	Upper 95% CI
Unhealed stasis ulcer	0.633	0.149	18.015	<.0001	1.883	1.406	2.522
Healing surgical wound	−0.254	0.048	28.212	<.0001	0.776	0.706	0.852
Urinary incontinence in past 14 days	0.161	0.077	4.367	0.037	1.175	1.010	1.367
Urinary catheter	0.220	0.101	4.771	0.029	1.246	1.023	1.517
Severe bowel incontinence	0.206	0.070	8.725	0.003	1.228	1.072	1.408
Respiratory symptoms	0.175	0.075	5.404	0.020	1.191	1.028	1.380
Moderate short of breathing (Ref: no breathing problem)	0.145	0.049	8.915	0.003	1.156	1.051	1.272
Severe short of breathing (Ref: no breathing problem)	0.270	0.073	13.529	0.000	1.310	1.134	1.512
1 to 2 Depression symptoms	0.152	0.046	10.889	0.001	1.164	1.064	1.275
Functional Status							
Unable to bath self	0.106	0.045	5.613	0.018	1.112	1.019	1.214
Unable to ambulation	0.135	0.048	8.023	0.005	1.145	1.043	1.257
Unable eating by self	0.172	0.078	4.905	0.027	1.188	1.020	1.383
Degree of needing assistance with IADLs (severity bet. 9-11)	0.153	0.045	11.475	0.001	1.166	1.067	1.274
Degree of needing assistance with IADLs (severity bet. 12-15)	0.226	0.051	19.904	<.0001	1.253	1.135	1.384
Unbalance that Could Cause Fall	0.143	0.039	13.738	0.000	1.153	1.070	1.244
Medication information							
Taking 5 or more medications	0.161	0.044	13.508	0.000	1.174	1.078	1.280
Need assistance with injectable medication	0.212	0.055	14.880	0.000	1.236	1.110	1.376
Degree of medication assistance needed	0.083	0.017	23.137	<.0001	1.087	1.051	1.124
Vital Sign							
Pulse normal (ref: pulse abnormal)	−0.334	0.060	31.374	<.0001	0.716	0.637	0.805
Temperature normal (ref: abnormal)	−0.295	0.085	12.077	0.001	0.745	0.631	0.879
Temperature unknown (ref: abnormal)	−0.255	0.109	5.505	0.019	0.775	0.626	0.959

factors shown in Table 2 are the statistically significant (p < .05) variables selected by the stepwise logistic model with corresponding parameter estimates and odds ratios. The model was created a second time using the validation sample and found to be very similar to the original model. Results from the validation sample are available from the authors.

Using the predicted values from the logistic model and by reviewing the distribution of scores, seven risk categories were defined: very low (0.000-0.042), low (0.043-0.079), low-moderate (0.080-0.124), moderate (0.125-0.211), moderate-high (0.212-0.357), high (0.358-0.442) and very high (0.443-1.000). Table 3 shows a breakdown by risk level, the proportion of patients that had a hospitalization for the model development, validation and overall samples. As can be seen in the Table the model was equally effective in identifying patients at risk in the model development and validation samples.

The final set of analyses focused on validating whether the predicted risk scores based on the seven levels agreed with clinical judgments of risk using a similar 7-point scale. Cohen's kappa statistics were calculated

TABLE 3. Percentage of Patients Hospitalized by Risk Level

Based on	Risk Group	% Had Hospitalization
Modeling Data Set	Very Low	1.3
	Low	5.2
	Low-Mod	9.8
	Moderate	16.6
	Mod-High	28.8
	High	39.6
	Very High	49.5
Validation Data Set	Very Low	3.1
	Low	5.0
	Low-Mod	9.9
	Moderate	16.2
	Mod-High	28.7
	High	40.5
	Very High	51.3
Combined Data Sets	Very Low	2.2
	Low	5.1
	Low-Mod	9.8
	Moderate	16.4
	Mod-High	28.7
	High	40.0
	Very High	50.4

separately for each the clinicians that rated the blinded medical records. For "Clinician A" kappa was 0.52 and "Clinician B" kappa was 0.77, representing moderate to high inter-rater agreement.

DISCUSSION

An important goal in home health care is delivering targeted care that could potentially prevent a patient from being hospitalized. The risk model developed in the current study was designed to help home health care providers more effectively focus on patients that are at risk and to intervene appropriately. At minimum the risk model could be used by clinicians so that they are cued into addressing problems before the patient deteriorates to the stage where a hospital admission is unavoidable.

Overview of the Findings

Although the risk model is most effective when all of the weighted factors are combined for individual patients, general trends do emerge from information that is readily available at the time of intake and can be used in developing care plans. The data indicated that patients who had a previous history of home health care, emergent care or hospitalization and a high number of certified visits were at higher risk for hospitalization. Moreover, persons coming from an inpatient setting are likely to return to that setting.

Functional status at start of care was moderately predictive of risk, with the degree of IADL assistance being the most predictive. The potential for falling was also predictive. It appears that persons taking more than five medications and having difficulty managing the medications may need focused interventions to keep them out of the hospital. Given Happ et al's. (1997) findings on non-adherence contributing to hospitalization of patients with CHF, it is not surprising that inability to manage medications increases risk.

By far the strongest predictors of hospitalization were clinical factors. Individuals that had unhealed pressure or stasis ulcers, urinary incontinence, urinary catheters, respiratory symptoms, shortness of breath and depression were more likely to be in the higher risk groups, as were those with four or more diagnoses and those who had one of the top diagnoses (CHF, ischemic heart disease, diabetes with a wound complication, HIV/AIDS, renal failure) at entry into care. Basic information on vital signs at start of care was an important indicator of risk. For example, having a normal pulse and temperature significantly reduced the risk of hospitalization.

All of these results suggest that the complexity and severity of illness, as well as the specific conditions that could often trigger a hospitalization, should be considered when developing care plans for patients. As in previous research (D' Agostino et al., 1999), the current study found a diagnosis of CHF to be strongly related to hospitalization. Similarly, Vinson, Rich, Sperry, Shah and McNamara (1990) reviewed a sample of 161 elderly CHF patients and found that in almost 50% of the cases rehospitalization could have been avoided if patients were identified as high risk shortly after admission to home health care. Both of these studies point out that risk assessment and early intervention can help to prevent poor outcomes. Examples of recommendations for the treatment include consideration of remote physiological monitoring interventions, provision of extra services during the first two weeks of home care and use of critical pathways (Hoskins, Walton-Moss, Clark, Schroeder & Thiel, 1999).

A reassuring finding was that the amount of certified nursing, home health aide and social work visits were significant predictors of hospitalization. This suggests that clinicians were aware of the complexity of patients that could be at risk for hospitalization at the point when they are working with physicians to develop appropriate plans of care. There were other factors that could have alerted clinicians that patients were at risk for hospitalization as they were providing treatment to the patient: pressure and stasis ulcers not healing, respiratory problems, depression, inability to independently bathe, ambulate, feed/eat and manage medications and unsteadiness that could cause a fall. However, it is difficult to know based on the data available whether the clinicians were aware of these problems. The risk model could be helpful to clinicians by warning them about specific patients who potentially have important clinical issues that need to be addressed.

Application of the Risk Model

One of the most important findings of the current study was the high level of agreement between the risk model and clinical judgment. Anecdotal comments from clinicians suggested that the model includes the factors that are important and it identifies patients they would have classified as at risk. Based on the feedback, which confirmed that clinicians would accept the data, we began providing risk scores as part of a pilot at the end of 2005. Between 48 to 72 hours after information is gathered on a patient, clinicians receive an email or can go you an Intranet Web Site to view risk scores and individual predictors for patients that have recently started care. See Figure 1 for an example of the email sent each day to clinicians. We are currently testing whether providing the risk scores can assist clinicians in making decisions related to care planning. For example, clinicians are utilizing various approaches to avoiding hospitalizations including: front loading visits during the first weeks of care, ordering remote physiological monitors and seeking the assistance of an Advanced Practice Nurse (APN) for patients with a moderate-high to very high risk. Interventions such as integrating the APN into the care process, have been found to be very effective in reducing the rate of hospitalization (Brooten et al., 2002) and will probably be more valuable with higher risk patients. In addition, we are investigating providing the risk scores at point of care, via tablet computers that are already used by clinicians in the field. Hopefully, real time access will help prevent hospitalizations within the first few days of home health care.

Study Limitations

The model developed shows great promise but the findings should be viewed in light of the study's limitations. First, the model predicts hospitalizations but does not specifically identify those that are preventable. Second, the sample was selected from patients that had complete assessment data at start of care from only one agency. Therefore, the potential

FIGURE 1. Example of Email Alert Sent to Clinicians

From: tom.smith@vnsny.org
Sent: Friday, October 13, 2006 4:54 PM
Subject: Hospitalization Risk Email Alert

The following patients were recently admitted. Please review the risk sores. Clink on the risk levels to see scores on individual risk factors.

Case Number	Patient Name	Admit Date	Risk Level
9999999	TC	10/10/2006	Low-Mod
9999888	JM	10/10/2006	Low-Mod
9999777	RN	10/10/2006	Low-Mod
9999786	AD	10/10/2006	Mod-High
9999892	SM	10/10/2006	Mod-High
9999787	CR	10/10/2006	Low-Mod
9999000	NM	10/10/2006	High
9999120	TY	10/10/2006	Low

for selection bias exists and the results may not generalize to the broader population of home care recipients. Third, the model did not take into consideration mortality and patients hospitalized after discharge when classifying individuals into risk groups. Fourth, the model included a limited number of primary diagnoses as predictors of hospitalization. It is possible that other conditions and secondary diagnoses could be useful measures of illness severity. Lastly, since only start of care information was used in the model it may not apply when patients are re-certified.

CONCLUSIONS

Further research should replicate these findings at other home health agencies, explore whether risk assessment can improve clinical decision-making and to assess the impact on patient outcomes. Consideration should also be given to conducting analyses of predictors within specific diagnoses (e.g., CHF, diabetes, COPD). Nonetheless, the results of this study provide insight into the factors that could be used to identify patients who are at risk for hospitalization and can be used as a foundation for future studies and improvements in care. Clearly at the start of care it is possible to distinguish high risk patients that may need additional or different types of services. Quality improvement efforts could be implemented to target these patients to assess the feasibility and practicality of reducing hospitalizations.

NOTE

[1]The sample is based on episodes of care and is not a unique patient count because patients may have received care more than once during the study period.

REFERENCES

Anderson, M.A., Helms, L.B., Hanson, K.S. & DeVilder, N.W. (1999). Unplanned hospital readmissions: A home care perspective. *Nursing Research, 48(6)*, 299-307.
Boult, L., Boult, C., Pirie, P., & Pacala, J.T. (1994). Test-retest reliability of a questionnaire that identifies elders at risk for hospital admission. *Journal of the American Geriatric Society, 42(7)*, 707-11.
Brooten, D., Naylor, M.D., York, R., Brown, L.P., Munro, B.H., Hollingsworth, A.O., Cohen, S.M., Flinkler, S., Deatrcik, J. & Youngblut, J.M. (2002). Lessons learned from testing the quality cost model of advanced practice nursing (APN) transitional care. *Journal of Nursing Scholarship, 34(4)*, 369-375.
Coleman, E.A.,Wagner, E.H., Grothaus, L.C., Hecht, J., Savarino, J., & Buchner, D.M. (1998). Predicting hospitalization and functional decline in older health

plan enrollees: Are administrative data as accurate as self-report? *Journal of the American Geriatric Society, 46(4)*, 534-5.

Centers for Medicare and Medicaid Services (2002). *Outcome-Based Quality Improvement (OBQI): Implementation Manual.* Retrieved on December 27, 2006 from http://www.cms.hhs.gov/HomeHealthQualityInits/16_HHQIOASISOBQI.asp.

Centers for Medicare and Medicaid Services (2006). *Risk-adjusted Home Health Outcome Report.* Retrieved on December 27, 2006 from http://www3.cms.hhs.gov/apps/hha/hhaqi_start.asp.

Coleman, E.A., Min, S., Chomiak, A. & Kramer, A. M. (2004). Posthospital care transitions: Patterns, complications and risk identification, *Health Services Research, 39(5)*, 1449-1466.

D'Agostino, R.S., Jacobson, J., Clarkson, M., Svensson, L.G., Williamson, C. & Shahian, D.M. (1999). Readmission after cardiac operations: Prevalence, patterns, and predisposing factors. *Journal of Thoracic Cardiovascular Surgery, 118(5)*, 823-832.

Gautam, P., Macduff, C., Brown, I. & Squair, J. (1996). Unplanned readmissions of elderly patients. *Health Bulletin, 54(6)*, 449-457.

Happ, M.B., Naylor, M.D., & Roe-Prior, P. (1997). Factors contributing to rehospitalization of elderly patients with heart failure. *Journal of Cardiovascular Nursing, 11(4)*, 75-84.

Hoskins, L.M., Walton-Moss, B., Clark, H.M., Schroeder, M.A. & Thiel, L. Sr. (1999). Predictors of hospital readmission among the elderly with congestive heart failure. *Home Healthcare Nurse, 17(6)*, 373-381.

Humphrey, C.J. (2005). Pay-for-performance is coming to home care. *Home Healthcare Nurse, 23(4)*, 202.

Kliebsch, U., Siebert, H. & Brenner, H. (2000). Extent and determinants of hospitalization in a cohort of older disabled people. *Journal of the American Geriatric Society, 48(3)*, 289-294.

Rosati, R.J., Huang, L., Navaie-Waliser, M. & Feldman, P. H. (2003). Risk Factors for repeated hospitalizations among home health care recipients, *Journal for Healthcare Quality, 25*, 4-11.

Schwarz, K.A. (2000). Predictors of early hospital readmissions of older adults who are functionally impaired. *Journal of Gerontological Nursing, 26(6)*, 29-36.

Shaughnessy, P.W., Hittle, D.F., Crisler, K.S., Powell, M.C., Richard, A.A., Kramer, A.M., Schlenker, R.E., Steiner, J.F., Donelan-McCall, N.S., Beaudry, J.M., Mulvey-Lawlor, K.L. & Engle, K. (2002). Improving patient outcomes of home health care: Findings from two demonstration trials of outcome-based quality improvement, *Journal of the American Geriatric Society, 50(8)*, 1456-7.

Vinson, J.M., Rich, M.W., Sperry, J.C., Shah, A.S., & McNamara, T. (1990). Early readmission of elderly patients with congestive heart failure. *Journal of the American Geriatric Society, 38(12)*, 1290-1295.

Wagner, J.T., Bachmann, L.M., Boult, C., Harari, D., von Renteln-Kruse, W., Egger, M., Beck, J.C. & Stuck, A. E. (2006). Predicting the risk of hospital admission in older persons: Validation of a brief self-administered questionnaire in three European countries, *JAGS, 54*, 1271–1276.

doi:10.1300/J027v26n04_03

Bouncing-Back: Rehospitalization in Patients with Complicated Transitions in the First Thirty Days After Hospital Discharge for Acute Stroke

Amy J. H. Kind, MD
Maureen A. Smith, MD, MPH, PhD
Nancy Pandhi, MD, MPH
Jennifer R. Frytak, PhD
Michael D. Finch, PhD

Amy J.H. Kind is affiliated with the Department of Population Health Sciences, and the Department of Medicine, Geriatrics Division, University of Wisconsin School of Medicine and Public Health, Madison, WI. She is also affiliated with the William S. Middleton Hospital, Geriatric Research Education and Clinical Center, United States Department of Veterans Affairs, Madison, WI. Maureen A. Smith is affiliated with the Department of Population Health Sciences, University of Wisconsin School of Medicine and Public Health, Madison, WI. Nancy Pandhi is affiliated with the Department of Population Health Sciences and the Department of Family Medicine, University of Wisconsin School of Medicine and Public Health, Madison, WI. Jennifer R. Frytak is affiliated with i3 Innovus, Eden Prairie, MN. Michael D. Finch is affiliated with the Center for Health Care Policy and Evaluation, Eden Prairie, MN.

Address correspondence to: Dr. Amy J. H. Kind, William S. Middleton VA Hospital–GRECC, 2500 Overlook Terrace, Madison, WI 53705 (E-mail: ajk@medicine.wisc.edu).

This study was supported by a grant (R01-AG19747) from the National Institute of Aging (Principal Investigator: Maureen Smith, MD PhD).

[Haworth co-indexing entry note]: "Bouncing-Back: Rehospitalization in Patients with Complicated Transitions in the First Thirty Days after Hospital Discharge for Acute Stroke." Kind, Amy J. H. et al. Co-published simultaneously in *Home Health Care Services Quarterly*® (The Haworth Press, Inc.) Vol. 26, No. 4, 2007, pp. 37-55; and: *Charting a Course for High Quality Care Transitions* (ed: Eric A. Coleman) The Haworth Press, Inc., 2007, pp. 37-55. Single or multiple copies of this article are available for a fee from The Haworth Document Delivery Service [1-800-HAWORTH, 9:00 a.m. - 5:00 p.m. (EST). E-mail address: docdelivery@haworthpress.com].

SUMMARY. *Background:* "Bounce-backs" (movements from a less intensive to a more intensive care setting) soon after hospital discharge are common, but reasons for bouncing-back remain unknown.

Objective: To examine how the primary diagnosis for first rehospitalization relates to thirty-day bounce-back number and initial discharge destination in acute stroke.

Population: Administrative data from 5,250 Medicare beneficiaries ≥ 65 years discharged with acute ischemic stroke in 1998-2000 to a rehabilitation center, skilled nursing facility or home with home health care and with at least one thirty day rehospitalization.

Analysis: Probability of thirty-day bounce-back was calculated using multivariate models.

Results: Infections and aspiration pneumonitis were the most common reasons for rehospitalization, regardless of initial discharge site.

Conclusions: Efforts addressing aspirations and infections, the preventable complications of immobility, will be critical in decreasing acute stroke bounce-backs. doi:10.1300/J027v26n04_04 *[Article copies available for a fee from The Haworth Document Delivery Service: 1-800-HAWORTH. E-mail address:<docdelivery@haworthpress.com> Website: <http://www.HaworthPress.com> © 2007 by The Haworth Press, Inc. All rights reserved.]*

KEYWORDS. Transition, stroke, rehospitalization, aspiration, infection

INTRODUCTION

In the current system of specialized health care, patients with complex chronic health conditions like acute stroke often require care across multiple settings and experience numerous care transitions (Coleman, 2003). These patients are at risk for "bounce-backs" (i.e., "complicated transitions"), movement from a less intense to a more intense care setting (e.g., home to the hospital), soon after hospital discharge (Coleman, Min, Chomiak & Kramer, 2004). Stroke patients are at especially high risk for bouncing-back with 20% of acute stroke patients experiencing at least one bounce-back and 16% of those experiencing more than one bounce-back within thirty days of hospital discharge (Kind, Smith, Frytak & Finch, 2006). Many of these bounce-backs are to the hospital (Kind et al., 2006). A number of publications have examined factors influencing rehospitalization in acute stroke patients, including insurance type

(Smith, Frytak, Liou & Finch, 2005), clinician specialty (Goldstein, Matchar, Hoff-Lindquist, Samsa & Horner, 2003, Mitchell, Ballard, Whisnant, Ammering, Samsa & Matchar, 1996, Smith, Liou, Frytak & Finch, 2006), initial discharge destination (Kind et al., 2006), patient functional ability and race (Kind et al., 2006, Ottenbacher, Smith, Illig, Fiedler, Gonzales & Granger, 2001). Yet few studies have examined specific rehospitalization diagnoses in acute stroke patients (Smith et al., 2005, Smith et al., 2006) and no studies have examined how initial discharge destination or number of thirty day bounce-backs relate to these diagnoses. A better understanding of this relationship may allow for the development of strategies to prevent or predict bounce-backs in acute stroke patients.

The goal of this study is to examine how the primary diagnosis for initial rehospitalization relates to thirty-day bounce-back number and initial stroke hospitalization discharge destination in acute stroke patients.

METHODS

Population and Sampling

We identified 5,250 Medicare beneficiaries 65 years of age and older discharged alive with acute ischemic stroke to a rehabilitation center, skilled nursing facility/long-term care or home with home health care during, 1998-2000. Patients were from 11 metropolitan regions of the country (Smith et al., 2005) and had at least one rehospitalization in the first thirty days after discharge. Patients were included in the sample if they had an International Classification of Diseases, 9th edition (ICD-9) diagnosis code of 434 or 436 in the first position on the discharge diagnosis list from an acute care hospitalization, which has been found to accurately identify acute ischemic stroke in 89-90% of cases (Benesch, Witter, Wilder, Duncan, Samsa & Matchar, 1997). If a patient had more than one acute ischemic stroke discharge over the study period, one discharge was randomly selected. This approach did not require analyses accounting for repeated observations on the same patient.

We obtained health maintenance organization (HMO) data from a large national managed care organization and fee-for-service (FFS) data from the Centers for Medicare and Medicaid Services (CMS). Our sample included 570 HMO patients with acute ischemic stroke (from 422 hospitals) enrolled in 11 Medicare Plus Choice plans serving 93 metropolitan counties primarily in the eastern half of the United States.

Comparable data were obtained for 4,680 FFS patients discharged with acute ischemic stroke from the same hospitals. The Institutional Review Board at the University of Wisconsin approved this study.

Data Extraction

We obtained enrollment data and final institutional and physician/ supplier claims for all study patients from one year prior to their index hospital admission date to one year after their index hospital admission date. Both HMO and FFS patients had claims submitted using identical forms (Medicare/Medicaid Health Insurance Common Claim Form, 2002, National Uniform Billing Committee (NUBC), 1994). We also obtained all claims for HMO patients submitted to the HMO from out-of-network facilities. For all patients, we obtained the Medicare denominator file to determine age, gender, race, zip code, Medicaid enrollment and date of death. This file was used to exclude beneficiaries who had end-stage renal disease, were missing Medicare Part A or Part B coverage, or received railroad retirement benefits.

Variables

The main dependent variable was the primary diagnosis for the first rehospitalization within thirty days of discharge. Primary diagnoses for the first rehospitalization were categorized using Clinical Classification Software (Agency for Healthcare Research and Quality, 2003). The main explanatory variables were the number of bounce-backs within the first thirty days of acute stroke hospitalization and the acute stroke hospitalization discharge destination (i.e., rehabilitation center, skilled nursing facility or home with home health care). "Bounce-back" (i.e., complicated transition) was defined as movement from a less intense to a more intense care setting, with hospital being the most intense on the care spectrum, then emergency room (ER), followed by skilled nursing facility/rehabilitation center/long-term care, then home with home health care, and, finally, home without home health care as the least intense (Coleman et al., 2004).

We obtained initial discharge destination from facility and non-facility claims occurring within one day of index hospitalization discharge date. Using facility claims, we identified patients admitted to rehabilitation facilities (freestanding or inpatient unit) and skilled nursing facilities. We used the place of service code on subsequent physician claims to identify patients discharged to long-term care facilities. Remaining patients were categorized as either home with home care claims within thirty days after the stroke discharge date or home with no home care claims. Patients with ER visits or rehospitalization within thirty days of the index hospitalization discharge date were identified using subsequent facility claims. For each patient, all identified sites of care within thirty days of the index hospitalization discharge date were sequentially ordered by date of service. This ordering enabled examination for movement from a less intense to a more intense care setting (a bounce-back). Patients were grouped into categories of one bounce-back and survived thirty days, one bounce-back and died within thirty days, and more than one bounce-back for analysis. Additional stratifications were not performed as too few patients were present in the ≥ 3 bounce-back category to allow for analysis.

We included individual and neighborhood sociodemographic characteristics as control variables. Individual characteristics included age, gender, race, HMO membership and an indicator identifying beneficiaries with low to modest income who were fully enrolled in Medicaid or received some help with Medicare cost-sharing through Medicaid. Zip+4 data were used to link patient data to the corresponding Census, 2000 block group and to obtain neighborhood socioeconomic characteristics including percent over 24 years of age with college degree and percent below poverty line (Krieger, Williams & Moss, 1997).

Individual comorbidities, length of index hospital stay and measures of stroke severity were also included as control variables. We identified 30 comorbid conditions by incorporating information from the index hospitalization, all hospitalizations during the prior year, and all physician claims during the prior year using methods proposed by Elixhauser et al., (Elixhauser, Steiner, Harris & Coffey, 1998) and Klabunde et al. (Klabunde, Potosky, Legler & Warren, 2000). Of these 30 conditions, we included the 12 comorbidities present in over 5% of our sample as explanatory variables. We also coded the following: hospitalization during the year prior to the index hospitalization, dementia (Pippenger, Holloway & Vickrey, 2001), stroke during the year prior to the index hospitalization (Samsa, Bian, Lipscomb & Matchar, 1999), and concurrent cardiac events (acute myocardial infarction, unstable angina pectoris, coronary artery bypass graft and cardiac catheterization). Additionally, the Centers for Medicare and Medicaid Services hierarchical condition categories (CMS-HCC) score for the year prior to admission was calculated for each subject and included in models as a comprehensive risk adjustment measure (Pope, Kautter, Ellis, Ash, Ayanian, Lezzoni, Ingber, Levy & Robst, 2004). Two validated indicator variables, mechanical ventilation (CPT 94656, 94657; ICD-9 96.7x) (Horner, Sloane & Kahn, 1998) and placement or revision of a gastrostomy tube (CPT 43750,43760,43761,43832,43246; ICD-9 43.11) (Quan, Parsons & Ghali, 2004), were used to represent disease severity during index hospitalization.

Analysis

For each thirty day bounce-back number and initial discharge destination combination, adjusted predicted probabilities were calculated for the primary diagnosis of the first rehospitalization. Analyses were conducted using SAS version 8.0 (SAS Institute, 2002) and Stata version 7.0 (Stata Corporation, 1999). Results of analyses are reported in adjusted probabilities and 95% confidence intervals (CI). All confidence intervals and significance tests were significant at $p < 0.05$ and were calculated using robust estimates of the variance that allowed for clustering of patients within hospitals. Models included age (65-69 years, 70-74 years, 75-79 years, 80-85 years and 85+ years), gender, race (Caucasian, African American and Other), Medicaid, HMO membership, percentage of the census block group aged 25+ with college degrees, percentage of persons in the census block group below the poverty line, length of index hospital stay, prior hospitalization, prior stroke, cardiac arrhythmias, congestive heart failure, chronic pulmonary disease, uncomplicated diabetes mellitus, complicated diabetes mellitus, hypertension, fluid and electrolyte disorders, valvular disease, peripheral vascular disorders, hypothyroidism, solid tumor without metastasis, deficiency anemias, depression, dementia, concurrent cardiac event, other comorbidity count, CMS-HCC score, mechanical ventilation and presence of gastrostomy tube.

RESULTS

Population Characteristics

Table 1 provides key characteristics of the acute stroke population studied stratified by thirty day bounce-back category (i.e., one bounce-back and survived thirty days, one bounce-back and died within thirty days

TABLE 1. Key Characteristics of Rehospitalized Acute Stroke Patients by Bounce-Back Category (N = 5,250)*

Characteristic	One bounce-back, survived 30 days (N = 3,683)	One bounce-back, died 30 days (N = 671)	More than one bounce-back (N = 896)	p-value
Sociodemographic				
Age (mean in years)	80 (7)	83 (8)	81 (7)	<0.0001
Female	62	58	60	0.085
Caucasian	79	82	74	0.001
African-American	16	13	21	0.001
Other	4	4	5	0.001
Medicaid	20	23	22	0.103
HMO membership	11	9	12	0.160
		0.12	0.13	
% in block group below the poverty line (mean)	0.13 (0.12)	(0.12) 0.23	(0.12) 0.22	0.464
% adults > = 25 years in block group with college degre (mean)	0.23 (0.16)	(0.16)	(0.16)	0.207
Index Hospitalization				
		8.64	7.59	
Length of Stay in days (standard deviation)	6.83 (5.45)	(6.41)	(5.72)	<0.0001
Discharged from Index Hospital Stay to:				
Home with Home Health	24	11	25	
Rehabilitation Center	26	18	17	
Skilled Nursing Facility or Long-Term Care	50	71	58	
Prior medical history				
HCC Score Prior to Index Hospital Discharge	2.6 (1.34)	3.09 (1.43)	2.78 (1.47)	<0.0001
Prior hospitalization	48	52	53	0.018
Prior stroke	9	9	10	0.725
Cardiac arrhythmias	43	50	46	0.001

TABLE 1 (continued)

Characteristic	One bounce-back, survived 30 days (N = 3,683)	One bounce-back, died 30 days (N = 671)	More than one bounce-back (N = 896)	p-value
Congestive heart failure	31	39	31	<0.0001
Chronic pulmonary disease	22	30	25	<0.0001
Diabetes, uncomplicated	25	27	25	0.352
Diabetes, complicated	10	9	10	0.588
Hypertension	76	71	78	0.011
Fluid and electrolyte disorders	30	33	35	0.010
Valvular disease	19	19	19	0.944
Peripheral vascular disorders	17	20	17	0.094
Hypothyroidism	12	13	12	0.718
Solid tumor without metastasis	13	11	13	0.396
Deficiency anemias	18	21	22	0.002
Depression	11	11	9	0.428
Dementia	27	29	29	0.240
Concurrent cardiac event	2	3	3	0.528
Other comorbidity count	0.54 (0.79)	0.66 (0.84)	0.65 (0.86)	<0.0001
Disease severity				
Mechanical ventilation	2	5	3	<0.0001
Gastrostomy tube	12	29	15	<0.0001

* Values represent percents unless specified otherwise. Parentheses indicate standard deviations.

and more than one bounce-back). Those with more than one bounce-back within the first thirty days were significantly more likely than the other two bounce-back groups to be African American (21%), have hypertension (78%) and fluid and electrolyte disorders (35%). Stroke patients with one bounce-back who died within thirty days of acute stroke discharge were significantly more likely to be older (averaging 83 years old), have a longer acute stroke hospitalization length of stay (average 8.64 days), have congestive heart failure (39%) and chronic pulmonary disease (30%), have a higher HCC score, and were more apt to have been on mechanical ventilation (5%) and have had a gastrostomy tube (29%). They were less likely to be African American (13%). Stroke patients with one bounce-back who survived at least thirty days were generally younger and had fewer comorbidities. In all bounce-back groups the majority of stroke patients were initially discharged to skilled nursing facilities or long-term care. The group with one bounce-back who died within thirty days had the highest percentage of discharges to skilled nursing or long-term care facilities (71%).

Primary Diagnoses for First Rehospitalizations

Over the entire study sample, primary rehospitalization diagnoses differed slightly by bounce-back category (Table 2). Stroke patients with one bounce-back who survived thirty days and those with more than one bounce-back were most likely to be rehospitalized for infections and aspiration pneumonitis, both with adjusted probabilities of 23% and 95% CI of (21.24, 24.56) and (19.75, 25.76) respectively. However, when these groups were compared to stroke patients with one bounce-back who died within thirty days, the stroke patients who died were significantly more likely to be rehospitalized for infections and aspiration pneumonitis, with an adjusted probability of 38% (95% CI = 33.89-42.06). Heart disease was the second most common rehospitalization diagnosis for stroke patients with one bounce-back who survived thirty days and for those with multiple bounce-backs, both at 15%. For stroke patients with one bounce-back who died within thirty days, heart disease (12%), acute cerebrovascular disease (13%) and other respiratory and circulatory diseases (11%) were the next most common rehospitalization diagnoses.

Rehospitalization diagnoses differed depending upon the patient's acute stroke hospitalization discharge destination. Of acute stroke patients initially discharged home with home health care (Table 3), patients with one bounce-back who survived thirty days were most apt to be rehospitalized with infections and aspiration pneumonitis (21%), followed by heart disease (16%). For patients with more than one bounce-back initially discharged home with home health care, heart disease (20%) and infections/aspiration pneumonitis (15%) were also the most common rehospitalization diagnoses. Of stroke patients with one bounce-back who died within thirty days and who were initially discharged home with home health care, 30% of rehospitalizations were due to infections or aspiration pneumonitis, while 17% were secondary to acute cerebrovascular disease.

For stroke patients initially discharged to rehabilitation centers (Table 4), infections and aspiration pneumonitis were the most common rehospitalization diagnoses in all three bounce-back groups. For both

TABLE 2. Probabilities and 95% confidence intervals (CI) for the relationship between bounce-back category and primary diagnosis for first rehospitalization (N = 5,250)

Clinical Classification System (CCS)*	CCS Level	Frequency (N = 5,250)	One bounce-back, survived 30 days		More than one bounce-back		One bounce-back, died 30 days	
			Prob[†]	95 % CI	Prob[†]	95 % CI	Prob[†]	95 % CI
Infections and aspiration pneumonitis	1, 8.1, 9.1, 10.4.1, 12.1, 13.1	1,295	0.23	[0.2124, 0.2456]	0.23	[0.1975, 0.2576]	0.38	[0.3389, 0.4206]
Heart disease	7.2	301	0.15	[0.1370, 0.1642]	0.15	[0.1222, 0.1758]	0.12	[0.0972, 0.1502]
Acute cerebrovascular disease	7.3.1	168	0.08	[0.0674, 0.0882]	0.09	[0.0679, 0.1082]	0.13	[0.0964, 0.1546]
Non-acute cerebrovascular disease	7.3.2, 7.3.3, 7.3.4, 7.3.6	804	0.04	[0.0314, 0.0500]	0.03	[0.0220, 0.0466]	0.02	[0.0065, 0.0270]
Respiratory disease other than infection/aspiration and circulatory disease other than heart	7.1, 7.4, 7.5, 8.2, 8.3, 8.5, 8.6, 8.8, 8.9	261	0.08	[0.0728, 0.0920]	0.08	[0.0632, 0.1024]	0.11	[0.0808, 0.1349]
Symptoms, signs, and ill-defined conditions	17	429	0.03	[0.0231, 0.0376]	0.02	[0.0109, 0.0314]	0.01	[0.0017, 0.0257]
Injury and poisoning	16	478	0.06	[0.0553, 0.0742]	0.06	[0.0483, 0.0816]	0.02	[0.0099, 0.0302]
Other	Remaining codes	1,514	0.32	[0.3068, 0.3421]	0.33	[0.2994, 0.3652]	0.21	[0.1801, 0.2450]

* Category indicates primary diagnosis for first rehospitalization within 30 days of the index admission

[†] Adjusted for age, gender, race, Medicaid, HMO membership, % of the census block group aged 25+ with college degrees, % of persons in the census block group below the poverty line, length of index hospital stay, prior hospitalization, prior stroke, cardiac arrhythmias, congestive heart failure, chronic pulmonary disease, uncomplicated diabetes, complicated diabetes, hypertension, fluid and electrolyte disorders, valvular disease, peripheral vascular disorders, hypothyroidism, solid tumor without metastasis, deficiency anemias, depression, dementia, concurrent cardiac events, mechanical ventilation, gastrostomy tube, other comorbidity count and CMS/HCC score.

the surviving one bounce-back group and the multiple bounce-back group, heart disease was the next most common reason for rehospitalization, while acute cerebrovascular disease was the second most common diagnosis observed for the one bounce-back and died group (19%).

Finally, stroke patients initially discharged to skilled nursing or long-term care facilities (Table 5) also experienced infections and aspiration pneumonitis as the most common rehospitalization diagnoses. These particular diagnoses were significantly more common than all others

TABLE 3. Probabilities and 95% confidence intervals (CI) for the relationship between bounce-back category and primary diagnosis for first rehospitalization for stroke patients discharged home with home health care (N = 1,187)

Clinical Classification System (CCS)*	CCS Level	Frequency (N = 1,187)	One bounce-back, survived 30 days		More than one bounce-back		One bounce-back, died 30 days	
			Prob[†]	95 % CI	Prob[†]	95 % CI	Prob[†]	95 % CI
Infections and aspiration pneumonitis	1, 8.1, 9.1, 10.4.1, 12.1, 13.1	214	0.21	[0.1768, 0.2414]	0.15	[0.0953, 0.2002]	0.30	[0.2022, 0.4066]
Heart disease	7.2	66	0.16	[0.1303, 0.1828]	0.20	[0.1474, 0.2600]	0.08	[0.0161, 0.1526]
Acute cerebrovascular disease	7.3.1	52	0.10	[0.0752, 0.1205]	0.08	[0.0469, 0.1196]	0.17	[0.0725, 0.2670]
Non-acute cerebrovascular disease	7.3.2, 7.3.3, 7.3.4, 7.3.6	192	0.06	[0.0424, 0.0801]	0.05	[0.0233, 0.0830]	0.01	[−0.0114, 0.0344]
Respiratory disease other than infection/aspiration and circulatory disease other than heart	7.1, 7.4, 7.5, 8.2, 8.3, 8.5, 8.6, 8.8, 8.9	103	0.07	[0.0526, 0.0902]	0.09	[0.0567, 0.1313]	0.09	[0.0193, 0.1522]
Symptoms, signs, and ill-defined conditions	17	81	0.04	[0.0229, 0.0487]	0.02	[0.0038, 0.0414]	0.01	[−0.0092, 0.0283]
Injury and poisoning	16	135	0.06	[0.0470, 0.0823]	0.07	[0.0313, 0.1001]	0.01	[−0.0113, 0.0368]
Other	Remaining codes	344	0.30	[0.2694, 0.3376]	0.33	[0.2632, 0.3965]	0.32	[0.2101, 0.4337]

* Category indicates primary diagnosis for first rehospitalization within 30 days of the index admission
[†] Adjusted for age, gender, race, Medicaid, HMO membership, % of the census block group aged 25+ with college degrees, % of persons in the census block group below the poverty line, length of index hospital stay, prior hospitalization, prior stroke, cardiac arrhythmias, congestive heart failure, chronic pulmonary disease, uncomplicated diabetes, complicated diabetes, hypertension, fluid and electrolyte disorders, valvular disease, peripheral vascular disorders, hypothyroidism, solid tumor without metastasis, deficiency anemias, depression, dementia, concurrent cardiac events, mechanical ventilation, gastrostomy tube, other comorbidity count and CMS/HCC score

over all bounce-back categories. When comparing between bounce-back categories in this discharge group, patients with one bounce-back who died were significantly more likely to have diagnoses of infections and aspiration pneumonitis (43%) than their counterparts in the other two bounce-back categories.

Stroke patients surviving one bounce-back were very similar in their rehospitalization diagnoses to those with more than one bounce-back,

TABLE 4. Probabilities and 95% confidence intervals (CI) for the relationship between bounce-back category and primary diagnosis for first rehospitalization for stroke patients discharged to rehabilitation centers (N = 1,230)

Clinical Classification System (CCS)*	CCS Level	Frequency (N = 1,230)	One bounce-back survived 30 days		More than one bounce-back		One bounce-back, died 30 days	
			Prob†	95% CI	Prob†	95% CI	Prob†	95% CI
Infections and aspiration pneumonitis	1, 8.1, 9.1, 10.4.1, 12.1, 13.1	224	0.19	[0.1592, 0.2242]	0.24	[0.1543, 0.3186]	0.33	[0.2368, 0.4148]
Heart disease	7.2	63	0.20	[0.1694, 0.2332]	0.24	[0.1532, 0.3281]	0.16	[0.0973, 0.2300]
Acute cerebrovascular disease	7.3.1	42	0.07	[0.0561, 0.0905]	0.11	[0.0568, 0.1570]	0.19	[0.1222, 0.2556]
Non-acute cerebrovascular disease	7.3.2, 7.3.3, 7.3.4, 7.3.6	268	0.03	[0.0207, 0.0456]	0.03	[-0.0004, 0.0525]	0.01	[-0.0050, 0.0328]
Respiratory disease other than infection/aspiration and circulatory disease other than heart	7.1, 7.4, 7.5, 8.2, 8.3, 8.5, 8.6, 8.8, 8.9	56	0.08	[0.0634, 0.1026]	0.06	[0.0206, 0.1042]	0.10	[0.0492, 0.1547]
Symptoms, signs, and ill-defined conditions	17	105	0.03	[0.0196, 0.0466]	0.01	[-0.0048, 0.0306]	0.01	[-0.0082, 0.0253]
Injury and poisoning	16	123	0.07	[0.0474, 0.0836]	0.03	[0.0023, 0.0645]	0.01	[-0.0082, 0.0260]
Other	Remaining codes	349	0.32	[0.2824, 0.3553]	0.28	[0.2010, 0.3614]	0.19	[0.1156, 0.2610]

* Category indicates primary diagnosis for first rehospitalization within 30 days of the index admission

† Adjusted for age, gender, race, Medicaid, HMO membership, % of the census block group aged 25+ with college degrees, % of persons in the census block group below the poverty line, length of index hospital stay, prior hospitalization, prior stroke, cardiac arrhythmias, congestive heart failure, chronic pulmonary disease, uncomplicated diabetes, complicated diabetes, hypertension, fluid and electrolyte disorders, valvular disease, peripheral vascular disorders, hypothyroidism, solid tumor without metastasis, deficiency anemias, depression, dementia, concurrent cardiac events, mechanical ventilation, gastrostomy tube, other comorbidity count and CMS/HCC score.

regardless of discharge site. Confidence intervals for all diagnoses in these two bounce-back groups overlap.

DISCUSSION

In summary, infections and aspiration pneumonitis were the most common reasons for rehospitalization in stroke patients with at least one bounce-back to the hospital in the first thirty days after acute

TABLE 5. Probabilities and 95% confidence intervals (CI) for the relationship between bounce-back category and primary diagnosis for first rehospitalization for stroke patients discharged to a skilled nursing facility or long-term care (N = 2,833)

Clinical Classification System (CCS)*	CCS Level	Frequency (N = 2,833)	One bounce-back, survived 30 days		More than one bounce-back		One bounce-back, died 30 days	
			Prob†	95% CI	Prob†	95% CI	Prob†	95% CI
Infections and aspiration pneumonitis	1, 8.1, 9.1, 10.4.1, 12.1, 13.1	857	0.25	[0.2334, 0.2743]	0.26	[0.2225, 0.3058]	0.43	[0.3812, 0.4744]
Heart disease	7.2	172	0.13	[0.1151, 0.1474]	0.10	[0.0677, 0.1224]	0.11	[0.0825, 0.1436]
Acute cerebrovascular disease	7.3.1	74	0.07	[0.0595, 0.0850]	0.09	[0.0576, 0.1129]	0.09	[0.0602, 0.1184]
Non-acute cerebrovascular disease	7.3.2, 7.3.3, 7.3.4, 7.3.6	344	0.04	[0.0267, 0.0468]	0.03	[0.0162, 0.0458]	0.02	[0.0049, 0.0317]
Respiratory disease other than infection/aspiration and circulatory disease other than heart	7.1, 7.4, 7.5, 8.2, 8.3, 8.5, 8.6, 8.8, 8.9	102	0.09	[0.0726, 0.0984]	0.08	[0.0569, 0.1098]	0.11	[0.0810, 0.1478]
Symptoms, signs, and ill-defined conditions	17	243	0.03	[0.0176, 0.0348]	0.02	[0.0086, 0.0371]	0.02	[0.0017, 0.0302]
Injury and poisoning	16	220	0.06	[0.0499, 0.0769]	0.07	[0.0487, 0.0964]	0.02	[0.0103, 0.0377]
Other	Remaining codes	821	0.33	[0.3070, 0.3545]	0.35	[0.2968, 0.3947]	0.20	[0.1590, 0.2355]

* Category indicates primary diagnosis for first rehospitalization within 30 days of the index admission

† Adjusted for age, gender, race, Medicaid, HMO membership, % of the census block group aged 25+ with college degrees, % of persons in the census block group below the poverty line, length of index hospital stay, prior hospitalization, prior stroke, cardiac arrhythmias, congestive heart failure, chronic pulmonary disease, uncomplicated diabetes, complicated diabetes, hypertension, fluid and electrolyte disorders, valvular disease, peripheral vascular disorders, hypothyroidism, solid tumor without metastasis, deficiency anemias, depression, dementia, concurrent cardiac events, mechanical ventilation, gastrostomy tube, other comorbidity count and CMS/HCC score.

stroke hospitalization, regardless of the initial discharge site. However, infections and aspiration pneumonitis accounted for significantly more rehospitalizations in the group with one bounce-back who died within the first thirty days, and tended to account for more rehospitalizations for acute stroke patients initially discharged to skilled nursing facilities. Rehospitalizations for acute cerebrovascular disease were most common in the group with one bounce-back who died within thirty days of acute stroke hospitalization. Surviving one bounce-back stroke patients were very similar in their rehospitalization diagnoses to those with more than one bounce-back, regardless of discharge site.

Aspiration pneumonitis and infections are critically important diagnoses in acute stroke patients and one of the most common reasons for stroke mortality after hospitalization (Aslanyan, Weir, Diener, Kaste & Lees, 2004). It is well accepted that complications of immobility, like aspiration pneumonia and infections, account for as many as 51% of stroke deaths in the first thirty days (Bernhardt, Dewey, Thrift & Donnan, 2004). Our findings that these diagnoses were the primary reasons for bounce-backs to the hospital, therefore, agree well with the previous stroke literature in this regard. The high mortality rates accompanying aspiration pneumonia (Aslanyan et al., 2004) likely also accounted for its significantly higher representation in the one bounce-back and died within thirty days category of patients. Overall, this particular bounce-back group was sicker with higher comorbidity burden and greater numbers of gastrostomy tubes. Gastrostomy tubes have high aspiration pneumonia complication rates (James, Kapur & Hawthorne, 1998). The high rate of gastrostomy tube use in the one bounce-back and died group likely at least partially accounts for the significant percentage of rehospitalizations for aspiration pneumonitis/infections in this particular group. By understanding the importance of aspirations and infections in stroke patient rehospitalization, strategies may be designed to prevent these conditions and, thus, potentially decrease bounce-backs.

We demonstrated that aspirations and infections caused the majority of rehospitalizations in skilled nursing and long-term care facility stroke patients. As these diagnoses are often the result of immobility (Bernhardt et al., 2004, Stroke Unit Trialists' Collaboration (SUTC), 1997), they should be preventable to some degree. Stroke patients in skilled nursing and long-term care facilities may provide an excellent target group for universal aspiration pneumonitis and infection prevention efforts. Previous studies have demonstrated that neurology specialty and stroke unit care during an acute stroke hospitalization may decrease a stroke patient's subsequent risk for rehospitalization with infection or aspiration pneumonia, likely through the increased ordering of early mobilization and swallowing consultations (Smith et al., 2006, Stroke Unit Trialists' Collaboration (SUTC), 1997). Targeted dysphagia programs, in particular, have been shown to substantially reduce pneumonia rates (Doggett, Tappe, Mitchell, Chapell, Coates & Turkelson, 2001). Further investigation into aspiration and infection prevention in acute stroke patients, and universal implementation of these preventive efforts in high risk settings, like skilled nursing and long-term care facilities, is needed.

Although infections and aspiration pneumonitis accounted for the majority of rehospitalizations in skilled nursing, long-term care and rehabilitation facility patients, each of these settings is well equipped to treat such medical disorders on-site, when not severe. Additionally, existing literature suggests an improved outcome for patients treated on-site (Dosa, 2005).While our data do not allow us to comment on medical appropriateness, it is reasonable to assume that some proportion of the observed rehospitalizations could have been treated on-site and, therefore, represent preventable bounce-backs. Unfortunately, the existing U.S. health system incentive structure does not encourage on-site care for medical conditions that could be treated equally well in either the present sub-acute care setting or the hospital. There is little to no financial benefit and potential medical-legal risk to treating such patients on-site. Modifications to this incentive structure will play a critical role in any health policy strategy to reduce bounce-back rates.

The similarity of rehospitalization diagnoses regardless of initial discharge site supports the idea that post-acute care services may be interchangeable. However, this "interchangeability" concept remains controversial. Previous studies utilizing Medicare administrative data have supported the idea of interchangeability by noting that the choice of post-acute care service type depends more on region, availability and reimbursement form than on other factors (Buntin, Garten, Paddock, Saliba, Totten & Escarce, 2005, Kane, Lin & Blewett, 2002, Lin, Kane, Mehr, Madsen & Petroski, 2006). However, a number of stroke specific studies have found inpatient rehabilitation to result in superior patient outcomes when compared to other post-acute care settings (Deutsch, Granger, Heinemann, Fiedler, DeJong, Kane, Ottenbacher, Naughton & Trevisan, 2006, Kind et al., 2006, Kramer, Steiner, Schlenker, Eilertsen, Hrincevich, Tropea, Ahmad & Eckhoff, 1997). Continued research, including prospective randomized controlled trials, will be necessary before this debate reaches resolution.

Recurrent strokes were more strongly represented as a primary reason for rehospitalization in stroke patients with one bounce-back who died, than in any other bounce-back category. In patients with a previous ischemic stroke the 5 year risk for recurrent fatal stroke is 3.7% (Dhamoon, Sciacca, Rundek, Sacco & Elkind, 2006). However, within the first thirty days after an initial ischemic stroke, recurrent stroke has been demonstrated to cause 14% of all deaths (de Jong, van Raak, Kessels &

Lodder, 2003). Our results agree well with the prior literature in this regard. Prevention of recurrent stroke provides another important way of potentially decreasing bounce-backs in acute stroke patients.

The stroke group with one bounce-back who survived thirty days and the group with multiple bounce-backs exhibited very similar rehospitalization diagnostic profiles. No one diagnostic category seems to differentiate stroke patients with multiple bounce-backs from those with one bounce-back. This finding supports the position that factors other than disease type, such as difficult to measure socioeconomic factors or patient choice, may be leading to multiple bounce-backs. Previous research examining predictors of bouncing-back demonstrated that African American race, in particular, was the strongest risk factor for multiple bounce-backs (Kind et al., 2006). Additional research examining patients with multiple bounce-backs is needed to fully understand, and thus prevent, this costly phenomenon.

This study has limitations. To address the potential problems associated with administrative diagnosis and procedure codes, we used codes previously shown to accurately identify ischemic stroke (Benesch et al., 1997). Nevertheless, in any study utilizing administrative data some misclassification may occur (McGlynn, Damberg, Kerr & Brook, 1998). Since patients with stroke documentation in the non-primary diagnostic position have greater comorbidity burden and 30-day mortality, by using the primary discharge diagnosis code we may have biased the sample toward more benign outcomes (Tirschwell & Longstreth, 2002). However, our use of the primary diagnosis code probably enabled us to avoid problems that might have been brought about by "up-coding," an intensive coding methodology sometimes utilized by health systems to maximize revenue, since up-coding most likely affects secondary diagnoses. Our measures of stroke severity were limited but valid (Horner et al., 1998, Quan et al., 2004). However, in the absence of more definitive severity measures, such as post-stroke functional status, it is impossible to comment on the appropriateness of patient discharge from the index hospitalization. Additionally, administrative data provides no direct measures of patient preference. Stroke patients' preferences, especially regarding code status, likely influence their chance of experiencing bounce-backs and, possibly, rehospitalizations (Zweig, Kruse, Binder, Szafara & Mehr, 2004). Thus, lack of information regarding patient preference is a major limitation of this particular research approach. Finally, it is unclear whether these findings would apply to non-stroke populations. Further study of bounce-backs in patient populations other than acute stroke is needed.

In conclusion, our research has a number of broad implications. Aspiration pneumonitis and infections are the most important reasons for thirty day rehospitalization in acute stroke patients. Prevention efforts specifically targeting populations at high risk for these complications of immobility, like skilled nursing or long-term care facility patients, may prove extremely valuable in decreasing bounce-backs in stroke patients. Additionally, changes to the existing financial and medical-legal health system incentive structure for treating patients on-site will likely be critical in decreasing bounce-back rates. Recurrent stroke is another important reason for bounce-backs in acute stroke patients, especially for patients who die within thirty days of acute stroke hospitalization. Prevention of recurrent stroke provides another important way to potentially decrease bounce-back number, and possibly thirty day mortality, in acute stroke patients. Finally, since surviving stroke patients with one bounce-back and those with multiple bounce-backs do not differ significantly in their rehospitalization diagnoses, it is possible that non-medical unmeasured factors, such as patient culture or choice, drive recurrent bounce-backs.

REFERENCES

Agency for Healthcare Research and Quality. Clinical Classifications Software (ICD-9-CM): Summary and Downloading Information [computer program]. Rockville, MD: Agency for Healthcare Research and Quality; 2003.

Aslanyan, S., Weir, C. J., Diener, H.-C., Kaste, M., & Lees, K. R. (2004). Pneumonia and urinary tract infection after acute ischaemic stroke: A tertiary analysis of the GAIN International trial. *Eur J Neurol, 11*(1), 49-53.

Benesch, C., Witter, D. M., Jr., Wilder, A. L., Duncan, P. W., Samsa, G. P., & Matchar, D. B. (1997). Inaccuracy of the International Classification of Diseases (ICD-9-CM) in identifying the diagnosis of ischemic cerebrovascular disease. *Neurology, 49*(3), 660-664.

Bernhardt, J., Dewey, H., Thrift, A., & Donnan, G. (2004). Inactive and alone: Physical activity within the first 14 days of acute stroke unit care. *Stroke, 35*(4), 1005-1009.

Buntin, M. B., Garten, A. D., Paddock, S., Saliba, D., Totten, M., & Escarce, J. J. (2005). How much is postacute care use affected by its availability? *Health Serv Res, 40*(2), 413-434.

Coleman, E. A. (2003). Falling through the cracks: Challenges and opportunities for improving transitional care for persons with continuous complex care needs. *J Am Geriatr Soc, 51*(4), 549-555.

Coleman, E. A., Min, S. J., Chomiak, A., & Kramer, A. M. (2004). Posthospital care transitions: Patterns, complications, and risk identification. *Health Serv Res, 39*(5), 1449-1465.

de Jong, G., van Raak, L., Kessels, F., & Lodder, J. (2003). Stroke subtype and mortality. A follow-up study in 998 patients with a first cerebral infarct. *J Clin Epidemiol, 56*(3), 262-268.

Deutsch, A., Granger, C. V., Heinemann, A. W., Fiedler, R. C., DeJong, G., Kane, R. L., Ottenbacher, K. J., Naughton, J. P., & Trevisan, M. (2006). Poststroke rehabilitation: Outcomes and reimbursement of inpatient rehabilitation facilities and subacute rehabilitation programs. *Stroke, 37*(6), 1477-1482.

Dhamoon, M. S., Sciacca, R. R., Rundek, T., Sacco, R. L., & Elkind, M. S. (2006). Recurrent stroke and cardiac risks after first ischemic stroke: The Northern Manhattan Study. *Neurology, 66*(5), 641-646.

Doggett, D. L., Tappe, K. A., Mitchell, M. D., Chapell, R., Coates, V., & Turkelson, C. M. (2001). Prevention of pneumonia in elderly stroke patients by systematic diagnosis and treatment of dysphagia: An evidence-based comprehensive analysis of the literature. *Dysphagia, 16*(4), 279-295.

Dosa, D. (2005). Should I hospitalize my resident with nursing home-acquired pneumonia? *J Am Med Dir Assoc, 6*(5), 327-333.

Elixhauser, A., Steiner, C., Harris, D. R., & Coffey, R. M. (1998). Comorbidity measures for use with administrative data. *Med Care, 36*(1), 8-27.

Goldstein, L. B., Matchar, D. B., Hoff-Lindquist, J., Samsa, G. P., & Horner, R. D. (2003). VA Stroke Study: Neurologist care is associated with increased testing but improved outcomes. *Neurology, 61*(6), 792-796.

Horner, R. D., Sloane, R. J., & Kahn, K. L. (1998). Is use of mechanical ventilation a reasonable proxy indicator for coma among Medicare patients hospitalized for acute stroke? *Health Serv Res, 32*(6), 841-859.

James, A., Kapur, K., & Hawthorne, A. B. (1998). Long-term outcome of percutaneous endoscopic gastrostomy feeding in patients with dysphagic stroke. *Age Ageing, 27*(6), 671-676.

Kane, R. L., Lin, W. C., & Blewett, L. A. (2002). Geographic variation in the use of post-acute care. *Health Serv Res, 37*(3), 667-682.

Kind, A. J. H., Smith, M., Frytak, J., & Finch, M. (2006). Bouncing-back: Patterns and predictors of complicated transitions thirty days after hospitalization for acute stroke. *J Am Geriatr Soc,* (in press).

Klabunde, C. N., Potosky, A. L., Legler, J. M., & Warren, J. L. (2000). Development of a comorbidity index using physician claims data. *J Clin Epidemiol, 53*(12), 1258-1267.

Kramer, A. M., Steiner, J. F., Schlenker, R. E., Eilertsen, T. B., Hrincevich, C. A., Tropea, D. A., Ahmad, L. A., & Eckhoff, D. G. (1997). Outcomes and costs after hip fracture and stroke. A comparison of rehabilitation settings. *JAMA, 277*(5), 396-404.

Krieger, N., Williams, D. R., & Moss, N. E. (1997). Measuring social class in US public health research: concepts, methodologies, and guidelines. *Annu Rev Public Health, 18,*341-378.

Lin, W. C., Kane, R. L., Mehr, D. R., Madsen, R. W., & Petroski, G. F. (2006). Changes in the use of postacute care during the initial Medicare payment reforms. *Health Serv Res, 41*(4), 1338-1356.

McGlynn, E. A., Damberg, C. L., Kerr, E. A., & Brook, R. H. (1998). *Health information systems: design issues and analytic applications.* Santa Monica: RAND.

Medicare/Medicaid Health Insurance Common Claim Form, Instructions and Supporting Regulations. Form No. CMS-1500, CMS-1490U, CMS-1490S (OMB #0938-0008). 2002.

Mitchell, J. B., Ballard, D. J., Whisnant, J. P., Ammering, C. J., Samsa, G. P., & Matchar, D. B. (1996). What role do neurologists play in determining the costs and outcomes of stroke patients? *Stroke, 27*(11), 1937-1943.

National Uniform Billing Committee (NUBC). Form UB-92: American Hospital Association; 1994.

Ottenbacher, K. J., Smith, P. M., Illig, S. B., Fiedler, R. C., Gonzales, V., & Granger, C. V. (2001). Characteristics of persons rehospitalized after stroke rehabilitation. *Arch Phys Med Rehabil, 82*(10), 1367-1374.

Pippenger, M., Holloway, R. G., & Vickrey, B. G. (2001). Neurologists' use of ICD-9CM codes for dementia. *Neurology, 56*(9), 1206-1209.

Pope, G. C., Kautter, J., Ellis, R. P., Ash, A. S., Ayanian, J. Z., Lezzoni, L. I., Ingber, M. J., Levy, J. M., & Robst, J. (2004). Risk adjustment of Medicare capitation payments using the CMS-HCC model. *Health Care Financ Rev, 25*(4), 119-141.

Quan, H., Parsons, G. A., & Ghali, W. A. (2004). Validity of procedure codes in International Classification of Diseases, 9th revision, clinical modification administrative data. *Med Care, 42*(8), 801-809.

Samsa, G. P., Bian, J., Lipscomb, J., & Matchar, D. B. (1999). Epidemiology of recurrent cerebral infarction: A Medicare claims-based comparison of first and recurrent strokes on 2-year survival and cost. *Stroke, 30*(2), 338-349.

SAS Institute. SAS Statistical Software. 8.2 ed. Cary, NC: SAS Institute; 2002.

Smith, M. A., Frytak, J. R., Liou, J. I., & Finch, M. D. (2005). Rehospitalization and survival for stroke patients in managed care and traditional Medicare plans. *Med Care, 43*(9), 902-910.

Smith, M. A., Liou, J., Frytak, J. R., & Finch, M. D. (2006). 30-day survival and rehospitalization for stroke patients according to physician specialty. *Cerebrovasc Dis,* (accepted with minor revisions).

Stata Corporation. Stata Statistical Software. 8.0 ed. College Station, TX: Stata Corporation; 1999.

Stroke Unit Trialists' Collaboration (SUTC). (1997). How do stroke units improve patient outcomes? A collaborative systematic review of the randomized trials. *Stroke, 28*(11), 2139-2144.

Tirschwell, D. L. & Longstreth, W. T., Jr. (2002). Validating administrative data in stroke research. *Stroke, 33*(10), 2465-2470.

Zweig, S. C., Kruse, R. L., Binder, E. F., Szafara, K. L., & Mehr, D. R. (2004). Effect of do-not-resuscitate orders on hospitalization of nursing home residents evaluated for lower respiratory infections. *J Am Geriatr Soc, 52*(1), 51-58.

doi:10.1300/J027v26n04_04

Care Coordination
for Cognitively Impaired Older Adults
and Their Caregivers

Mary D. Naylor, PhD, RN, FAAN
Karen B. Hirschman, PhD, MSW
Kathryn H. Bowles, PhD, RN
M. Brian Bixby, MSN, CRNP, CS
JoAnne Konick-McMahan, RN, MSN, CCRN
Caroline Stephens, MSN, APRN, BC

SUMMARY. Dementia and delirium, the most common causes of cognitive impairment (CI) among hospitalized older adults, are associated with higher mortality rates, increased morbidity and higher health care costs. A growing body of science suggests that these older adults and

Mary D. Naylor is Marian S. Ware Professor in Gerontology and the Director of the Center for Health Transitions; Karen B. Hirschman is Research Assistant Professor; Kathryn H. Bowles is Associate Professor; M. Brian Bixby is Advance Practice Nurse; and JoAnne Konick-McMahan is Advance Practice Nurse; all affiliated with the School of Nursing, at the University of Pennsylvania. Caroline Stephens is a Predoctoral Student at the University of California, San Francisco.

Address correspondence to: Dr. Mary Naylor, Marian S. Ware Professor in Gerontology, University of Pennsylvania School of Nursing, Ralston House, 3615 Chestnut Street, Philadelphia, PA 19104 (E-mail: naylor@nursing.upenn.edu).

Funding for the projects presented in this manuscript were provided by the Alzheimer's Association, Chicago, IL, the Marian S. Ware Alzheimer Program at the University of Pennsylvania, and the National Institute on Aging (NIA, 5R01AG023116-02).

[Haworth co-indexing entry note]: "Care Coordination for Cognitively Impaired Older Adults and Their Caregivers." Naylor, Mary D. et al. Co-published simultaneously in *Home Health Care Services Quarterly®* (The Haworth Press, Inc.) Vol. 26, No. 4, 2007, pp. 57-78; and: *Charting a Course for High Quality Care Transitions* (ed: Eric A. Coleman) The Haworth Press, Inc. 2007, pp. 57-78. Single or multiple copies of this article are available for a fee from The Haworth Document Delivery Service [1-800-HAWORTH, 9:00 a.m. - 5:00 p.m. (EST). E-mail address: docdelivery@haworthpress.com].

Available online at http://hhc.haworthpress.com
doi:10.1300/J027v26n04_05

their caregivers are particularly vulnerable to systems of care that either do not recognize or meet their needs. The consequences can be devastating for these older adults and add to the burden of hospital staff and caregivers, especially during the transition from hospital to home. Unfortunately, little evidence exists to guide optimal care of this patient group. Available research findings suggest that hospitalized cognitively impaired elders may benefit from interventions aimed at improving care management of both CI and co-morbid conditions but the exact nature and intensity of interventions needed are not known. This article will explore the need for improved transitional care for this vulnerable population and their caregivers. doi:10.1300/J027v26n04_05 *[Article copies available for a fee from The Haworth Document Delivery Service: 1-800-HAWORTH. E-mail address: <docdelivery@haworthpress.com> Website: <http://www. HaworthPress.com> © 2007 by The Haworth Press, Inc. All rights reserved.]*

KEYWORDS. Dementia, delirium, transitional care, advanced practice nurses

BACKGROUND

For more than 15 years, our multidisciplinary research team has been testing evidence-based clinical interventions guided by the Quality Cost Model of APN Transitional Care (hereafter referred to as the APN Care Model). These interventions have been designed to improve the quality of care and outcomes of high risk cognitively intact older adults as they make the difficult transition from hospital to home. Findings from three NIH-funded randomized control trials (RCTs) have consistently demonstrated improved quality and reductions in hospital readmissions and health care costs among intervention patients compared to control patients receiving standard care (Naylor et al., 1994; Naylor et al., 1999; Naylor et al., 2004). Recently, our team has begun to extend application of the APN Care Model to other high risk patient groups. With the support of the Alzheimer's Association, we have conducted pilot studies that have yielded important information about the unique health issues faced by cognitively impaired older adults and their caregivers during transitions from hospitals to home and suggested the value of interventions designed specifically to meet their needs (Naylor, Stephens, Bowles, & Bixby, 2005). Currently, with the support of the National Institute of Aging and Marian S. Ware Alzheimer's Program, our team is testing a range of interventions designed to enhance the care management of elders with cognitive impairment (CI) and their caregivers throughout episodes of acute illnesses. The purpose of this paper is to examine the need for enhanced transitional care among hospitalized cognitively impaired older adults and their caregivers and to describe the evolution of a major research initiative designed to inform critically needed changes in clinical practices.

SIGNIFICANCE

Dementia and delirium are the two most common cognitive disorders affecting older adults and often coexist within this population. Dementia is a neurodegenerative disease characterized by memory impairment, other cognitive deficits and associated behavioral disorders that result in a progressive loss of autonomy in common daily activities (Caltagirone, Perri, Carlesimo, & Fadda, 2001). In contrast, delirium, an acute disruption in cognition characterized by disturbances in consciousness, orientation, memory, thought, perception and behavior, is a multi-factorial syndrome resulting from the interaction of patient vulnerability and hospital related insults (Inouye, 1994). At the time of hospital admission, between 15% and 20% of older adults meet the criteria for delirium-prevalent cases (Francis, Martin, & Kapoor, 1990; Cameron, Thomas, Mulvihill, & Bronheim, 1987; Erkinjuntti, Wikstrom, Palo, & Autio, 1986; S. Levkoff, Cleary, Liptzin, & Evans, 1991; Rockwood, 1989; Schor et al., 1992). Most studies report a subsequent incidence during hospitalization of 5% to 10% (Francis et al., 1990; Cameron et al., 1987; Erkinjuntti et al., 1986; Levkoff et al., 1991; Rockwood, 1989; Schor et al., 1992; Inouye, 1998). The prevalence of dementia among persons discharged from acute care hospitals ranges from 4% to 27% (Fick, Agostini, & Inouye, 2002). Prevalence rates for both conditions are expected to increase as the population ages (Caltagirone et al., 2001). Recent advances in science support a strong relationship between these cognitive disorders. Between one-quarter to three quarters of patients with delirium have dementia (Cole, 2004; Fick et al., 2002) and the presence of dementia increases the risk of delirium by fivefold (Elie, Cole, Primeau, & Bellavance, 1998). Therefore assessment of both delirium and dementia should be part of a comprehensive assessment at hospital admission and throughout the hospital stay.

Current evidence reveals a higher level of comorbidity among patients with CI than among cognitively intact patients (Fields, MacKenzie,

Charlson, & Sax, 1986; Gutterman, Markowitz, Lewis, & Fillit, 1999; Hill et al., 2002; Lyketsos, Sheppard, & Rabins, 2000; McCormick et al., 2001). Collectively, CI and chronic medical illnesses result in greater morbidity, increased preventable hospitalizations and poorer survival (Feil, Marmon, & Unutzer, 2003; Zuccala et al., 2003). Investigators hypothesize that medical conditions may negatively impact cognition and neurodegeneration (Bynum et al., 2004; Doraiswamy, Leon, Cummings, Marin, & Neumann, 2002; Feil et al., 2003; McCormick et al., 1994; Zuccala et al., 2003). Conversely, CI among elders with other comorbid conditions may lead to inaccurate symptom reporting, delayed or inadequate treatment of the comorbid conditions and nonadherence with prescribed therapies (Doraiswamy et al., 2002; McCormick et al., 1994; Sloan, Trogdon, Curtis, & Schulman, 2004; Sullivan-Marx, 1994). When CI co-exists with depression (approximately 20% of cases), adherence with prescribed therapies, and thus outcomes, are especially poor (Feil et al., 2003).

Despite its clinical importance, CI is often not detected or it is misdiagnosed (Francis, 1992; Francis & Kapoor, 1992; Gustafson et al., 1991; Inouye, 1994; Kakuma et al., 2003; Levkoff, Besdine, & Wetle, 1986; Rothschild, Bates, & Leape, 2000; Schor et al., 1992; Naylor et al., 2005). Consequently, CI often triggers a cascade of undesirable adverse clinical events (ACEs) such as deconditioning, falls, malnutrition, and incontinence during hospitalization and immediately following discharge (Fick & Foreman, 2000; Greenwald et al., 1989; Inouye, 1994; Muehrer, 2002; Rothschild et al., 2000). Even when assessed, CI among hospitalized elders is poorly managed. Management of symptoms (Burgener & Twigg, 2002; Wing, Phelan, & Tate, 2002), especially pain (Given & Given, 1991; Rothschild et al., 2000), is compromised and disruptive, unsafe behaviors are common and often untreated (Burgener & Twigg, 2002; Sullivan-Marx, 1994; Wing et al., 2002). Thus, delirium and dementia appear to be independently associated with significant increases in functional disability, numbers of hospitalizations, lengths of hospital stay, rates of admissions to nursing homes, rates of death and health care costs (Britton & Russell, 2001; Fick & Foreman, 2000; Francis et al., 1990; Inouye, 1994; Inouye, Rushing, Foreman, Palmer, & Pompei, 1998; Inouye, Schlesinger, & Lydon, 1999; Levkoff et al., 1992; Marcantonio, Flacker, Michaels, & Resnick, 2000; O'Keeffe & Lavan, 1997). In 1999, increased hospital admissions and longer lengths of stay accounted for greater than 50% of adjusted costs with admissions for preventable hospitalization, more than two times greater than for non-demented patients (Bynum et al., 2004). Delirium complicates stays accounted for an additional $6 billion (in 2000 U.S. dollars) of total Medicare expenditures (The Hospital Elder Life Program, 2003).

Most of the interventions reported to date have evaluated the effectiveness of early detection and management of causal factors of delirium. Study findings suggest that such approaches are modestly effective in preventing delirium among surgical patients (Gustafson et al., 1991; Inouye, Bogardus et al., 1999; Marcantonio, Flacker, Wright, & Resnick, 2001; Milisen et al., 2001; Wanich, Sullivan-Marx, Gottlieb, & Johnson, 1992). The few successful interventions targeting the management of delirium or dementia included training clinicians to improve the recognition and management of CI, using evidence-based clinical guidelines, and tailoring interventions to meet individualized needs (Inouye, Bogardus et al., 1999; Rizzo et al., 2001; Marcantonio et al., 2001; Young & George, 2003). Despite the fact that delirium can persist for months following discharge and both cognitive disorders continue to complicate the care of these patients following discharge, none of the reported interventions spanned hospital to home (Bogardus et al., 2003).

Often, it is left to family caregivers to meet the complex needs of cognitively impaired elders following hospital discharge. Study findings suggest that their lack of knowledge and skills contribute to poor patient outcomes (Kelley, Buckwalter, & Maas, 1999; Mui, 1995; Zarit, Reever, & Bach-Peterson, 1980), increased caregiver burden (Charlesworth, Riordan, & Sthepstone, 2000; Nolan, Grant, & Keady, 1996) and depression (Poulshock & Deimling, 1984). A meta-analysis of 30 studies testing psychosocial interventions for caregivers of people with dementia revealed that interventions that were more intensive, adapted to meet individualized needs, and targeted both patients and their caregivers were more successful in reducing caregiver burden, increasing their knowledge and skills, enhancing their satisfaction and preventing or delaying elders' institutionalization (Brodaty, Green, & Koschera, 2003).

In summary, CI is a major health problem complicating the care of increasing numbers of older adults hospitalized for an acute medical or surgical condition. Dementia and delirium, the most common causes of CI among these elders, are associated with higher mortality rates, increased morbidity and higher health care costs. A growing body of science suggests that these patients and their caregivers are particularly vulnerable to systems of care that either do not recognize or are unable to meet their needs. The consequences are devastating for the patients and their caregivers and add tremendous burden to hospital staffs coping with shortages of nurses. Thus, it is not surprising that the Institute of Medicine (IOM) identified improved care coordination of this patient group as a national priority for action (Institute of Medicine, 2003). Unfortunately, little evidence is available to guide optimal care of this patient group or to address the unique needs of their caregivers. Collectively, available evidence suggests that these patients may benefit from interventions aimed at improving management of CI, comorbid conditions or both but the exact nature and intensity of interventions needed to effectively and efficiently improve their outcomes and those of their caregivers is not known.

EXTENDING THE APN CARE MODEL TO COGNITIVELY IMPAIRED HOSPITALIZED ELDERS: BUILDING ON THE SCIENCE

Building on this base of science we designed a study to determine how large a problem CI was among elders hospitalized for common medical and surgical conditions. This pilot work had two phases, the first phase (Pilot Study I) consisted of determining the presence of CI among hospitalized older adults and the second phase (Pilot Study II) consisted of interviewing a small subset of older adults and caregivers to identify their needs during the transitions from hospitals to home. Findings from these studies informed the design of a large scale RCT.

Pilot Study I–Defining the Problem

To assess the extent of impairment in this population, older adults hospitalized from home were sequentially screened for the presence of CI at three urban hospitals in the Philadelphia area. Hospitalized elders were eligible if they were ≥ 70 years old; English speaking; admitted for a common cardiovascular, respiratory, orthopedic or endocrine medical or surgical event; and had a primary caregiver, defined as a spouse, family member, partner or friend, who provided assistance with care. After meeting inclusion criteria subjects were screened for CI using the Mini-Mental State Examination (MMSE) (Folstein, Folstein, & McHugh, 1975) (scores of <24 on this 30 item scale were considered impaired), Brief Dementia Severity Rating Scale (BDSRS) (Clark & Ewbank, 1996), and the Confusion Assessment Method (CAM) (Inouye et al., 1990) (scored as the presence or absence of delirium). A detailed description of the screening process is presented elsewhere (Naylor et al., 2005).

Findings: Of the 145 hospitalized elders screened in this study, 35% (51/145) had some form of CI (Naylor et al., 2005). Among the group of elders with CI, 65% met the criteria for CI based solely on the screening instruments (i.e., no diagnoses of dementia or delirium noted in the chart), 18% had a preexisting diagnosis of dementia, and 18% had a pre-existing diagnosis of delirium. In-depth interviews with a sub-sample of these elders and their caregivers (5/51) revealed numerous unmet needs including managing and negotiating care with multiple providers, managing illness (e.g., identifying and managing physical and psychological symptoms, adhering with prescribed therapies, managing problem behaviors, and lack of awareness of community resources), and psychosocial support and coping (e.g., depression among patients and burden, depression, isolation and fear among caregivers) (Naylor et al., 2005).

Pilot Study II–Testing the Feasibility of the APN Care Model

Using the results from Pilot Study I (Naylor et al., 2005) and prior transitional care work with cognitively intact elders (Naylor et al., 1999; Naylor et al., 2004; Naylor et al., 1994) Pilot Study II was designed to: (1) test the effectiveness of the APN Care Model specifically designed for the needs of cognitively impaired adults and their caregivers; (2) determine which elements and interventions are most beneficial to cognitively impaired older adults and their caregivers during hospitalization and post-discharge periods; and, (3) design a large scale follow-up study to improve outcomes for hospitalized cognitively impaired older adults and caregivers.

Screening criteria and enrollment procedures were the same as in Pilot Study I. The sample of convenience consisted of 11 patient-caregiver dyads. All approached agreed to participate, one died during the index hospitalization. During each data collection visit (baseline, 2-, 6-, 12-weeks) several standardized instruments interviewer administered. In addition to the three CI screening scales–MMSE, BDSRS, and CAM–, data were collected on bothersome symptoms (Symptom Bother Scale) (Heidrich & Ryff, 1993), depression (Geriatric Depression Scale, GDS, and Center for Epidemiologic Studies Depression scale, CES-D) (Brink et al., 1982; Radloff, 1977), quality of life, assistance needed for activities of daily living, support provided by the caregiver, rehospitalizations, overall mental and physical health ratings, caregiver satisfaction, and patient behaviors.

Intervention: The intervention was specifically designed to make use of existing successful strategies shown to positively influence patient and caregiver outcomes. Patient-caregiver dyads received a six week APN provided transitional care intervention aimed at identifying and meeting the unique needs of the cognitively impaired older adult and their caregiver using the APN Care Model as a framework. The APNs were clinical nurse specialists or nurse practitioners with a Master of Science in Nursing specializing in adult health, acute care or gerontology with a minimum of 5 years experience post-Masters in the care of an elderly population. The specific nurses in this pilot had extensive experience with the application of the APN Care Model from previous work on the RCTs. The APNs acted as clinician and collaborator in acute care, rehabilitation or home settings performing a comprehensive physical, emotional, mental and social assessment and developing a unique plan of care working with the older adult, caregiver, and collaborating health care professionals to meet mutually agreed and attainable goals.

These APNs provided the vital link from one level of care to the home and in the home setting. They implemented a comprehensive plan of care through patient and caregiver education regarding diagnosis, symptom management, accessing needed services, equipment, and health care professionals. The nurse experts collaborated with primary care and specialist practitioners as well as other health care professionals to address needs and problems key to meeting goals and refining the plan of care to address changing patient and caregiver needs. The APNs focused on care coordination, advocacy, and education through home visits as well as phone contact to the older adult and provided demonstration of effective advocacy behavior for caregivers and other patient support.

RESULTS

Of the enrolled older adults, 5 were Caucasian and 5 African American; they ranged in age from 72-89 (mean 82.1±6.7 years) with a baseline mean MMSE score of 18 (±3.0; range 13-23). Caregivers were all female, aged 43-85 (mean 62); length of time in the caregiver role ranged from 1 month to 10.2 years. Four were Caucasian, 5 African American and 1 Native American. These women were primarily spouses or children of the care recipient (70%). Despite the challenges faced, they reported high self rated overall health scores and little desire to explore nursing home options. Sixty percent of the caregivers used no support services, yet all performed at least four care giving tasks; 30%

percent reported they had no one to help them and were also the primary caregiver to another person. When assessed for burden, 30% felt they were "missing out on life," 40% wished they could escape from their situation, 40% felt emotionally drained and 30% thought that "life would be different." Depression scores using the CES-D indicated high levels of depressive symptoms at baseline (Mean = 16±7; range 12-34). The most common behavioral problems reported by caregivers were auditory hallucinations and day/night disturbances.

CASE STUDIES

The following two case studies illustrate the application of the APN Care Model and the challenging situations and complex management encountered while caring for older adults with CI and their caregivers.

Case Study #1

Complexity of Care: On enrollment, Mr. S. had 10 co-morbid conditions requiring active treatment. These included: heart failure (HF) with an ejection fraction of <15% treated with deployment of a biventricular pacemaker, coronary artery disease (CAD) resulting in two prior coronary artery bypass grafting procedures and an angioplasty; ventricular tachycardia necessitating placement of an automatic internal cardioverter defibrillator (AICD); chronic renal insufficiency; anemia; benign prostate hypertrophy; depression treated with Paxil; dementia treated with Aricept; and bilateral cataract removal. He was prescribed 12 daily medications. His MMSE score was 16 at enrollment. During his inpatient episode Mr. S exhibited signs of hospital acquired delirium manifested by sleep disturbances, aggressive behavior towards staff and refusal of most basic care. Mr. S also reported being greatly bothered by a number of symptoms including aching, feeling tired and weak, pain, shortness of breath, incontinence, and concentration and memory problems.

Mr. S's available resources were his two daughters and wife. One daughter lived with the patient but was physically not available to assist, though she frequently told Mrs. S, her mother, what to do. This often made Mrs. S. resentful and not willing to give up "control" of care. Additionally, Mr. S. had a large circle of friends who called frequently but were not physically able to assist. The patient had friends at a senior center and, when well enough, visited on a weekly basis but was actively discouraged from attending by his wife. The living areas of the home were on one floor with limited steps at entrances. Mr. S changed to a new primary care provider (PCP) during hospitalization. In addition he had been seen as an outpatient by a nephrologist and three cardiologists.

Clinical Priorities: Mr. S had progressive congestive HF and required vigilant home monitoring. He did not tolerate the preferred heart failure treatments having an intolerance to angiotension converting enzyme (ACE) inhibitor and an "allergy" (rash) to Carvedilol. He had repeated hospitalizations for exacerbation of HF responsive to intravenous (IV) Milrinone. He was diagnosed with multi-infarct dementia by his former PCP after reported memory decline over the prior three years. Approximately six months prior to enrollment in this pilot he began treatment with Aricept. Mr. S's wife stated she saw improvement but his daughter noted little improvement but did indicate there was no continued memory decline. At discharge his new PCP was unfamiliar with the prior CI treatment and discontinued the Aricept Mr. S had been receiving, believing it was prescribed to treat the hospital acquired delirium not the underlying dementia. The new PCP believed the delirium would clear slowly on return to home and improve with congestive HF management.

Barriers: Barriers to implementation of the APN Care Model are multifaceted but typically issues are related to one or more of the following: the elder, the caregiver, the health system or communication. In this case study all four areas acted as barriers to implementation and needed to be addressed by the APN in order to achieve minimal success. Mr. S's diagnosis' of depression, dementia and delirium in the hospital resulted in limitations in recall, at times even not recognizing the APN or PCP, which affected the ability to provided meaningful patient education or an active role for the older adult in needs assessment and goal formation.

Conflicting goals and perceptions of the caregivers, their competing needs and grief over the potential loss of their loved one provided significant barriers for the APN. Mrs. S was depressed over her husband's rapid physical and mental decline over the past few weeks, stating she *"thought her life would be different at this point in time."* She was also highly anxious regarding care giving responsibilities frequently stating, *"I'm going to kill him if I don't do it right"* and *"My daughter makes me feel so guilty."* Mr. S's daughter was in denial of CI although acknowledging that her father could no longer tell time. The caregivers had been in family counseling to address mother-daughter relationship issues for 2 years. They stopped going to weekly sessions when Mr. S was hospitalized. The APN discussed the need to resume the family counseling and encouraged both to continue to seek counseling which they did. The caregivers were not physically or emotionally able to manage the home IV Milrinone which limited the cardiologist's treatment plan to optimizing oral HF medications.

Health systems issues impacted the implementation of the plan of care. The prior diagnosis of dementia made by a former PCP was not addressed by Mr. S's new provider and treatment with Aricept was discontinued. Treatment of his hospital acquired delirium was not addressed as the new PCP and family believed this would clear with Mr. S's return to a familiar environment and better management of HF. Additionally, the multiple specialist physicians involved in the case made contradictory recommendations regarding dementia treatment. One physician refused to continue Aricept as he thought there was a potential interaction with Coumadin and a potential heightened bleeding risk, another physician said the memory impairment, common in individuals with multiple CABG surgeries, was expected and not necessarily needing treatment while another physician weighed in that since the patient did not have Alzheimer's Disease, his antidepressant could be discontinued. This resulted in Mr. S exhibiting increased aggression and anger toward his family after discharge to home. The APN requested restarting the antidepressant with slow resolution of untoward behavior. Additionally, the APN sought referral to a memory disorder clinic. Given the long waiting list at a memory disorder clinic, referral to a geropsychiatric nurse practitioner was also sought and her insights were helpful in reinforcing the APNs recommendations and increasing physician-APN collaboration.

Facilitators: Facilitators to implementation of APN Care Model and attainment of patient and caregiver goals included: sufficient income, insurance and medication coverage; access to specialty and primary care; involvement of the area Alzheimer's Association; and positive supports from the visiting nurse association. Mr. S's MMSE scores improved over time from 16 to 21. In addition, Mr. S reported no longer being bothered by symptoms such as aching, pain, incontinence, and concentration problems. Despite these positives, the Mr. S's wife never felt comfortable with her care giving ability and Mr. S was admitted to a long term care facility after the sixth week of intervention.

Case Study #2

Complexity of Care: Mrs. J is an 86 year-old admitted to an outlying hospital for chest pain and shortness of breath. After initial stabilization she was transferred on day three of her hospitalization to a teaching hospital for further evaluation of her symptoms. After this transfer Mrs. J began to exhibit delirium—easy confusion, sleep disturbances, aggressive nighttime behaviors—without chronic mental status change which limited retention and ability to conduct necessary patient education. On enrollment, Mrs. J. had four co-morbid conditions: CAD requiring cardiac catheterization and placement of an intracoronary stent; arthritis; cataracts; and hypercholesterolemia. Her baseline MMSE score was 20. Mrs. J also reported being greatly bothered by feeling tired and achy.

Mrs. J lived alone and was her own primary caregiver. She was prescribed three medications on discharge. One medication was for short term use given the stent placement. The other medications were all new to Mrs. J as she had not previously taken daily standing medications. Resources available to Mrs. J included a niece who lived out of state (>4 hours travel) and a friend who lived near Mrs. J identified as helper and first contact. Mrs. J had not seen a doctor for checkups for many years and had many unmet preventative care needs. She was referred upon discharge to the PCP who had admitted her as well as the cardiologist who had seen her while hospitalized. She also identified a need for follow-up with an ophthalmologist to determine the status of her cataracts. Clinical priorities on discharge were monitoring of her liver enzymes which were elevated during hospitalization; diet education; development of an exercise program; clinical follow-up; medication education; and monitoring the recovery of her cognition.

Barriers: The primary barrier for Mrs. J was assuring safety during the transition to home on discharge and establishing a plan to monitor Mrs. J overnight during the first days after discharge. Given travel distances Mrs. J's niece could not actively participate in the provision of care. Mrs. J was able to identify friends who would be willing to assume this role for the short-term. Health system barriers included new providers; hospital acquired delirium with no medical or nursing notes to indicate this was assessed or being treated; lack of physical therapy consult despite a noted gait disturbance; and inadequate discharge planning assessment of needs related to transportation and clothing.

Facilitators: During the hospitalization nurses and physicians collaborated with the APN to assure transitional needs were met and safety at discharge was assured. This was accomplished through delay by one day, at the APNs suggestion, of Mrs. J's discharge home, identification of local caregivers able to spend the night at Mrs. J's home and assessment of Mrs. J's understanding of her CIand plan of care. The APN was able to visit Mrs. J within hours of her discharge and provide an in-depth assessment of her living conditions and trouble-shoot potential problems.

The APN was also able to work with the caregiver to educate her as to signs and symptoms to report and re-orientation strategies. The APN was flexible in scheduling visits to provide maximum support and assessment of the continuing delirium during the first two weeks of intervention.

In addition to these assets, Mrs. J had a prescription plan with minimal co-pay which was not a financial hardship. Her living arrangement was ideal, a first floor apartment with grab bars in bathroom, good lighting, laundry facilities on the same level and neighbors who checked on her daily. A friend assisted with laundry and visited daily after initially spending several nights at Mrs. J's home. Friends at the senior center were supportive through phone calls and visits. Another friend provided cleaning, transportation and food delivery. Importantly, Mrs. J trusted the APN, asked for help appropriately and followed through on directions about activities, medications, and diet. Though not physically present her niece seemed genuinely concerned via phone and asked appropriate questions. Through the intervention of the APN Mrs. J was able to return home after hospitalization avoiding short-term skilled nursing placement. During the course of the intervention Mrs. J's MMSE improved from 20 at enrollment to 28 at the 12 week follow up. Mrs. J also reported that the symptoms of feeling tired or achy no longer bothered her.

Overall Improvements Among All the Older Adults in the Pilot Study

Improvements in mean MMSE scores after six weeks of APN intervention (mean MMSE = 20.5) persisting to 12 weeks (mean MMSE = 22) post-enrollment were noted with most improvement in those older adults with a higher baseline MMSE. The nature and severity of symptom complaints were significantly reduced over the 12 week period (baseline Symptom Bother Scale–mean = 12.9 ± 7.4, range 3-22; 12 week follow up: mean = 8 ± 3.9, range 4-13) with particular improvements noted in management of pain and mobility.

Summary of Pilot Experience

Based on prior experience with similar high risk elders, the APNs provided valuable input related to the design and implementation of the pilot study intervention. For example, the APNs successfully identified nursing and medical champions at the sites who helped them influence the care of these older adults while hospitalized. In addition, they suggested the need for increased awareness by hospital staff about geropsychiatric resources for cognitively impaired patients and their caregivers. APNs reported little difficulty in tailoring the intervention to caregivers. All caregivers reported that they valued the involvement of the APN during the episode of illness. Finally, case studies completed by APNs highlighted the critical importance of interventions. Among nine older adults in the pilot, APNs prevented a serious medication error for one older adult and delayed discharges until essential follow-up care could be provided in the home for two other older adults, neither of whom had been identified by medical or nursing staff as having evidence of CI.

These pilot study findings coupled with the needs assessment revealed a high rate of unrecognized CI among hospitalized older adults and highlighted the unique needs and profound challenges facing elders and their caregivers as they adapt to a serious illness complicated by multiple comorbid conditions and CI. Improvements in mean MMSE scores at 12 week post-enrollment are likely the result of improvements or resolution of delirium. Findings informed the design of the intervention protocol, the APN orientation and training program, resource projections for the proposed study and modifications in data collection instruments.

DESIGNING A RESEARCH STUDY TO ADDRESS THE PROBLEM

With funding from the National Institute on Aging and the Marian S. Ware Alzheimer's Program we have designed an intervention study titled, "Hospital to Home: Cognitively Impaired Elders/Caregivers", to meet special needs of hospitalized elders with CI due to delirium, dementia or both. The interventions being tested in our current RCT were designed after synthesizing the published evidence and our own pilot findings. Our current work includes the strategies associated with positive results in the detection and management of CI and management of complex co-existing medication conditions during an acute episode of illness (Table 1).

Guided by Roy's Adaptation Model (Roy, 1976), a body of research in care management of cognitively intact high risk elders (Naylor et al., 1994; Naylor et al., 1999; Naylor et al., 2004), our pilot study findings (Naylor et al., 2005) and other empirical evidence, we developed

TABLE 1. Strategies Integrated into the Current RCT Interventions to Meet the Special Needs of Hospitalized Elders with Cognitive Impairment (CI) Due to Delirium, Dementia or Both

---

Strategies:

- Better screening and early detection of both delirium and dementia

- Prevention of adverse clinical events such as falls, drug interactions, incontinence

- Prevention of delirium

- Early diagnosis of delirium

- Measurement of depression

- Multi dimensional intervention (education, support, reorientation)

- Medication reviews

- Use of protocols and guidelines with hospital follow up and including both patients and their caregivers

- Tailoring interventions to meet the needs of the patients and caregivers

- Focus on recognition and management of CI, acute illness, and comorbid conditions

---

a research study to test different nurse models of care for cognitively impaired elders and their caregivers. The different models being tested are:

1. *Augmented Standard Care* (ASC)–Standard hospital and home care (if referred). Older adults receive an assessment for CI during the hospitalization through the use of standardized instruments; including a brief investigator developed 6-item orientation screen, the CLOX (Royall, Cordes, & Polk, 1998) and the Confusion Assessment Method (CAM) (Inouye et al., 1990). Immediate feedback from these screens is provided to patients' primary nurses, attending physicians and discharge planners is provided in the medical record by the subject screeners in the form of a note entered into the patient's medical record;

2. *Resource Nurse Care* (RNC)–Standard hospital and home care (if referred) plus early identification of CI during the older adult's hospitalization as is provided in ASC. In addition, these patients' hospital care will be reviewed by RNs trained in the use of expert clinical guidelines developed to enhance the care management of hospitalized cognitively impaired elders and to facilitate their transition from hospital to home; or,

3. *Advanced Practice Nurse Care* (APNC)–Standard hospital care, early identification of CI during the older adult's hospitalization, plus transitional (hospital to home) care substituting for standard home care and provided by masters prepared nurse specialists with advanced training in the management of cognitively impaired older adults using an evidence-based protocol designed specifically for this patient group and their caregivers. The APN is to be available by phone from 8:00AM-8:00PM Monday to Friday and 8:00AM–12:00PM on weekends to provide support for the older adult and family members as needed. For each older adult an individual plan is developed for care needs outside of these hours. Additionally, the APN has the flexibility to schedule visits at any time to best meet the needs of the older adult and caregiver.

To avoid cross contamination within sites each model of care will be tested at a different site. Then, we will compare across the three hospital sites the effects on health outcomes and costs of the interventions. Upon completion of this first part of the study, all three sites will enroll subjects and provide APNC. In the second part of the study, we will seek to confirm initial findings by comparing within each site and over time, the health and cost outcomes from patients treated with either ASC or RNC (both relatively lower intensity interventions) with the outcomes of patients at the same site observed after switching to APNC (a high intensity intervention). Outcome data for each part of the study will be collected at multiple intervals and extend through six months post-index hospital discharge. Findings have the potential to inform improved care management of these older adults and their caregivers, an IOM priority for national action (Institute of Medicine, 2003).

CONCLUSION

Cognitive impairment adds substantial complexity to care needs for older adults and strain on caregivers attempting to cope with these elders. The risk for adverse events, such as medication errors, increases with cognitive impairment. The current care system in the United States is inadequate to address needs of older adults with CI. This study has been substantially informed by our team's program of research conducted over the last 18 years and aimed at enhancing care coordination (Bowles, Foust, & Naylor, 2003; Bowles, Naylor, & Foust, 2002;

Bowles, 2000; Naylor, 2000, 2002; Naylor, Bowles, & Brooten, 2000; Naylor et al., 1999; Naylor et al., 2004; Naylor et al., 2005) and effective collaboration among physicians, nurses and other providers and communication with patients and their caregivers during critical transitions in care. Compared to standard care, findings from this body of research have consistently demonstrated the benefits of comprehensive APN-directed care in improving health outcomes and decreasing health care costs among high-risk cognitively intact elders making the difficult transition from hospital to home. Noteworthy are recent findings demonstrating the benefit of APN care on both the primary illness and comorbid conditions (Naylor et al., 2004). The need now is to apply this body of research to improving transitions in care for the growing population of cognitively impaired older adults and their caregivers.

REFERENCES

Bogardus, S. T., Jr., Desai, M. M., Williams, C. S., Leo-Summers, L., Acampora, D., & Inouye, S. K. (2003). The effects of a targeted multicomponent delirium intervention on postdischarge outcomes for hospitalized older adults. *Am J Med, 114*(5), 383-390. doi:10.1016/S0002-9343(02)01569-3

Bowles, K. H. (2000). Patient problems and nurse interventions during acute care and discharge planning. *J Cardiovasc Nurs, 14*(3), 29-41.

Bowles, K. H., Foust, J. B., & Naylor, M. D. (2003). Hospital discharge referral decision making: A multidisciplinary perspective. *Appl Nurs Res, 16*(3), 134-143. doi:10.1016/S0897-1897(03)00048-X

Bowles, K. H., Naylor, M. D., & Foust, J. B. (2002). Patient characteristics at hospital discharge and a comparison of home care referral decisions. *J Am Geriatr Soc, 50*(2), 336-342. doi:10.1046/j.1532-5415.2002.50067.x

Brink, T. L., Yesavage, J. A., Lum, O., Heersema, P. H., Adey, M., & Rose, T. L. (1982). Screening tests for geriatric depression. *Clinical Gerontologist, 1,* 37-43. doi:10.1300/J018v01n01_06

Britton, A., & Russell, R. (2001). Multidisciplinary team interventions for delirium in patients with chronic cognitive impairment. *Cochrane Database Syst Rev* (1), CD000395

Brodaty, H., Green, A., & Koschera, A. (2003). Meta-analysis of psychosocial interventions for caregivers of people with dementia. *J Am Geriatr Soc, 51*(5), 657-664. doi:10.1034/j.1600-0579.2003.00210.x

Burgener, S. C., & Twigg, P. (2002). Interventions for persons with irreversible dementia. *Annu Rev Nurs Res, 20,* 89-124.

Bynum, J. P., Rabins, P. V., Weller, W., Niefeld, M., Anderson, G. F., & Wu, A. W. (2004). The relationship between a dementia diagnosis, chronic illness, medicare expenditures, and hospital use. *J Am Geriatr Soc, 52*(2), 187-194. doi:10.1111/j.1532-5415.2004.52054.x

Caltagirone, C., Perri, R., Carlesimo, G. A., & Fadda, L. (2001). Early detection and diagnosis of dementia. *Arch Gerontol Geriatr Suppl, 7*, 67-75. doi:10.1016/S0167-4943(01)00122-4

Cameron, D. J., Thomas, R. I., Mulvihill, M., & Bronheim, H. (1987). Delirium: A test of the Diagnostic and Statistical Manual III criteria on medical inpatients. *J Am Geriatr Soc, 35*(11), 1007-1010.

Charlesworth, G., Riordan, J., & Sthepstone, L. (2000). Cognitive behavior therapy (CBT) for depressed carer of people with Alzheimer's disease and related disorders [Protocol]. *Cochrane Database Syst Rev, 3 (issue).*

Clark, C. M., & Ewbank, D. C. (1996). Performance of the dementia severity rating scale: A caregiver questionnaire for rating severity in Alzheimer disease. *Alzheimer Dis Assoc Disord, 10*(1), 31-39. doi:10.1097/00002093-199601010-00006

Cole, M. G. (2004). Delirium in elderly patients. *Am J Geriatr Psychiatry, 12*(1), 7-21. doi:10.1176/appi.ajgp.12.1.7

Doraiswamy, P. M., Leon, J., Cummings, J. L., Marin, D., & Neumann, P. J. (2002). Prevalence and impact of medical comorbidity in Alzheimer's disease. *J Gerontol A Biol Sci Med Sci, 57*(3), M173-177.

Elie, M., Cole, M. G., Primeau, F. J., & Bellavance, F. (1998). Delirium risk factors in elderly hospitalized patients. *J Gen Intern Med, 13*(3), 204-212. doi:10.1046/j.1525-1497.1998.00047.x

Erkinjuntti, T., Wikstrom, J., Palo, J., & Autio, L. (1986). Dementia among medical inpatients. Evaluation of 2000 consecutive admissions. *Arch Intern Med, 146*(10), 1923-1926. doi:10.1001/archinte.146.10.1923

Feil, D., Marmon, T., & Unutzer, J. (2003). Cognitive impairment, chronic medical illness, and risk of mortality in an elderly cohort. *Am J Geriatr Psychiatry, 11*(5), 551-560. doi:10.1176/appi.ajgp.11.5.551

Fick, D., & Foreman, M. (2000). Consequences of not recognizing delirium superimposed on dementia in hospitalized elderly individuals. *J Gerontol Nurs, 26*(1), 30-40.

Fick, D. M., Agostini, J. V., & Inouye, S. K. (2002). Delirium superimposed on dementia: A systematic review. *J Am Geriatr Soc, 50*(10), 1723-1732. doi:10.1046/j.1532-5415.2002.50468.x

Fields, S. D., MacKenzie, C. R., Charlson, M. E., & Sax, F. L. (1986). Cognitive impairment. Can it predict the course of hospitalized patients? *J Am Geriatr Soc, 34*(8), 579-585.

Folstein, M. F., Folstein, S. E., & McHugh, P. R. (1975). "Mini-mental state". A practical method for grading the cognitive state of patients for the clinician. *Journal of Psychiatric Research, 12*(3), 189-198. doi:10.1016/0022-3956(75)90026-6

Francis, J. (1992). Delusions, delirium, and cognitive impairment: The challenge of clinical heterogeneity. *J Am Geriatr Soc, 40*(8), 848-849.

Francis, J., & Kapoor, W. N. (1992). Prognosis after hospital discharge of older medical patients with delirium. *J Am Geriatr Soc, 40*(6), 601-606.

Francis, J., Martin, D., & Kapoor, W. N. (1990). A prospective study of delirium in hospitalized elderly. *Jama, 263*(8), 1097-1101.

Given, B. A., & Given, C. W. (1991). Family caregiving for the elderly. *Annu Rev Nurs Res, 9*, 77-101.

Greenwald, B. S., Kramer-Ginsberg, E., Marin, D. B., Laitman, L. B., Hermann, C. K., Mohs, R. C. et al. (1989). Dementia with coexistent major depression. *Am J Psychiatry, 146*(11), 1472-1478.

Gustafson, Y., Brannstrom, B., Berggren, D., Ragnarsson, J. I., Sigaard, J., Bucht, G. et al. (1991). A geriatric-anesthesiologic program to reduce acute confusional states in elderly patients treated for femoral neck fractures. *J Am Geriatr Soc, 39*(7), 655-662.

Gutterman, E. M., Markowitz, J. S., Lewis, B., & Fillit, H. (1999). Cost of Alzheimer's disease and related dementia in managed-medicare. *J Am Geriatr Soc, 47*(9), 1065-1071.

Heidrich, S. M., & Ryff, C. D. (1993). Physical and mental health in later life: The self-system as mediator. *Psychol Aging, 8*(3), 327-338. doi:10.1037/0882-7974. 8.3.327.

Hill, J. W., Futterman, R., Duttagupta, S., Mastey, V., Lloyd, J. R., & Fillit, H. (2002). Alzheimer's disease and related dementias increase costs of comorbidities in managed Medicare. *Neurology, 58*(1), 62-70.

Inouye, S. K. (1994). The dilemma of delirium: Clinical and research controversies regarding diagnosis and evaluation of delirium in hospitalized elderly medical patients. *Am J Med, 97*(3), 278-288. doi:10.1016/0002-9343(94)90011-6

Inouye, S. K. (1998). Delirium in hospitalized older patients. *Clin Geriatr Med, 14*(4), 745-764.

Inouye, S. K., Bogardus, S. T., Jr., Charpentier, P. A., Leo-Summers, L., Acampora, D., Holford, T. R. et al. (1999). A multicomponent intervention to prevent delirium in hospitalized older patients. *N Engl J Med, 340*(9), 669-676. doi:10.1056/ NEJM199903043400901

Inouye, S. K., Rushing, J. T., Foreman, M. D., Palmer, R. M., & Pompei, P. (1998). Does delirium contribute to poor hospital outcomes? A three-site epidemiologic study. *J Gen Intern Med, 13*(4), 234-242. doi:10.1046/j.1525-1497.1998.00073.x

Inouye, S. K., Schlesinger, M. J., & Lydon, T. J. (1999). Delirium: A symptom of how hospital care is failing older persons and a window to improve quality of hospital care. *Am J Med, 106*(5), 565-573. doi:10.1016/S0002-9343(99)00070-4.

Inouye, S. K., van Dyck, C. H., Alessi, C. A., Balkin, S., Siegal, A. P., & Horwitz, R. I. (1990). Clarifying confusion: the confusion assessment method. A new method for detection of delirium. *Ann Intern Med, 113*(12), 941-948.

Institute of Medicine. (2003). *Priority areas for national action: Transforming health care quality.* Washington, DC: National Academy Press.

Kakuma, R., du Fort, G. G., Arsenault, L., Perrault, A., Platt, R. W., Monette, J. et al. (2003). Delirium in older emergency department patients discharged home: Effect on survival. *J Am Geriatr Soc, 51*(4), 443-450. doi:10.1046/j.1532-5415.2003. 51151.x

Kelley, L. S., Buckwalter, K. C., & Maas, M. L. (1999). Access to health care resources for family caregivers of elderly persons with dementia. *Nurs Outlook, 47*(1), 8-14. doi:10.1016/S0029-6554(99)90036-2.

Levkoff, S., Cleary, P., Liptzin, B., & Evans, D. A. (1991). Epidemiology of delirium: An overview of research issues and findings. *Int Psychogeriatr, 3*(2), 149-167. doi:10.1017/S1041610291000625.

Levkoff, S. E., Besdine, R., & Wetle, T. (1986). Acute confusional stress (delirium) in the hospitalized elderly. In *Annual Review of Gerontology and Geriatrics* (Vol. 6, pp. 1-26). New York: Springer.

Levkoff, S. E., Evans, D. A., Liptzin, B., Cleary, P. D., Lipsitz, L. A., Wetle, T. T. et al. (1992). Delirium. The occurrence and persistence of symptoms among elderly hospitalized patients. *Arch Intern Med, 152*(2), 334-340. doi:10.1001/archinte.152.2.334

Lyketsos, C. G., Sheppard, J. M., & Rabins, P. V. (2000). Dementia in elderly persons in a general hospital. *Am J Psychiatry, 157*(5), 704-707. doi:10.1176/appi.ajp. 157.5.704.

Marcantonio, E. R., Flacker, J. M., Michaels, M., & Resnick, N. M. (2000). Delirium is independently associated with poor functional recovery after hip fracture. *J Am Geriatr Soc, 48*(6), 618-624.

Marcantonio, E. R., Flacker, J. M., Wright, R. J., & Resnick, N. M. (2001). Reducing delirium after hip fracture: A randomized trial. *J Am Geriatr Soc, 49*(5), 516-522. doi:10.1046/j.1532-5415.2001.49108.x.

McCormick, W. C., Hardy, J., Kukull, W. A., Bowen, J. D., Teri, L., Zitzer, S. et al. (2001). Healthcare utilization and costs in managed care patients with Alzheimer's disease during the last few years of life. *J Am Geriatr Soc, 49*(9), 1156-1160. doi:10.1046/j.1532-5415.2001.49231.x.

McCormick, W. C., Kukull, W. A., van Belle, G., Bowen, J. D., Teri, L., & Larson, E. B. (1994). Symptom patterns and comorbidity in the early stages of Alzheimer's disease. *J Am Geriatr Soc, 42*(5), 517-521.

Milisen, K., Foreman, M. D., Abraham, I. L., De Geest, S., Godderis, J., Vandermeulen, E. et al. (2001). A nurse-led interdisciplinary intervention program for delirium in elderly hip-fracture patients. *J Am Geriatr Soc, 49*(5), 523-532. doi:10.1046/j.1532-5415.2001.49109.x.

Muehrer, P. (2002). Research on co-morbidity, contextual barriers, and stigma: An introduction to the special issue. *J Psychosom Res, 53*(4), 843-845. doi:10.1016/ S0022-3999(02)00519-6.

Mui, A. C. (1995). Perceived health and functional status among spouse caregivers of frail older persons. *J Aging Health, 7*(2), 283-300.

Naylor, M., Brooten, D., Jones, R., Lavizzo-Mourey, R., Mezey, M., & Pauly, M. (1994). Comprehensive discharge planning for the hospitalized elderly. A randomized clinical trial. *Ann Intern Med, 120*(12), 999-1006.

Naylor, M. D. (2000). A decade of transitional care research with vulnerable elders. *J Cardiovasc Nurs, 14*(3), 1-14; quiz 88-19.

Naylor, M. D. (2002). Transitional care of older adults. *Annu Rev Nurs Res, 20*, 127-147.

Naylor, M. D., Bowles, K. H., & Brooten, D. (2000). Patient problems and advanced practice nurse interventions during transitional care. *Public Health Nurs, 17*(2), 94-102. doi:10.1046/j.1525-1446.2000.00094.x.

Naylor, M. D., Brooten, D., Campbell, R., Jacobsen, B. S., Mezey, M. D., Pauly, M. V. et al. (1999). Comprehensive discharge planning and home follow-up of hospitalized elders: A randomized clinical trial. *Jama, 281*(7), 613-620. doi:10.1001/jama. 281.7.613.

Naylor, M. D., Brooten, D. A., Campbell, R. L., Maislin, G., McCauley, K. M., & Schwartz, J. S. (2004). Transitional care of older adults hospitalized with heart failure: A randomized, controlled trial. *J Am Geriatr Soc, 52*(5), 675-684. doi:10.1111/j.1532-5415.2004.52202.x

Naylor, M. D., Stephens, C., Bowles, K. H., & Bixby, M. B. (2005). Cognitively impaired older adults: From hospital to home. *Am J Nurs, 105*(2), 52-61; quiz 61-52.

Nolan, M., Grant, G., & Keady, J. (1996). The Carers Act: Realising the potential. *Br J Community Health Nurs, 1*(6), 317-322.

O'Keeffe, S., & Lavan, J. (1997). The prognostic significance of delirium in older hospital patients. *J Am Geriatr Soc, 45*(2), 174-178.

Poulshock, S. W., & Deimling, G. T. (1984). Families caring for elders in residence: Issues in the measurement of burden. *J Gerontol, 39*(2), 230-239.

Radloff, L. S. (1977). The CES-D. Scale: A self-report depression scale for research on the general population. *Applied Psychological Measurement, 1*(3), 385-401.

Rizzo, J. A., Bogardus, S. T., Jr., Leo-Summers, L., Williams, C. S., Acampora, D., & Inouye, S. K. (2001). Multicomponent targeted intervention to prevent delirium in hospitalized older patients: What is the economic value? *Med Care, 39*(7), 740-752. doi:10.1097/00005650-200107000-00010.

Rockwood, K. (1989). Acute confusion in elderly medical patients. *J Am Geriatr Soc, 37*(2), 150-154.

Rothschild, J. M., Bates, D. W., & Leape, L. L. (2000). Preventable medical injuries in older patients. *Arch Intern Med, 160*(18), 2717-2728. doi:10.1001/archinte.160.18.2717.

Roy, C. (1976). *Introduction to nursing: An adaptation model.* Englewood Cliffs, NJ: Prentice-Hall.

Royall, D. R., Cordes, J. A., & Polk, M. (1998). CLOX: An executive clock drawing task. *J Neurol Neurosurg Psychiatry, 64*(5), 588-594.

Schor, J. D., Levkoff, S. E., Lipsitz, L. A., Reilly, C. H., Cleary, P. D., Rowe, J. W. et al. (1992). Risk factors for delirium in hospitalized elderly. *Jama, 267*(6), 827-831. doi:10.1001/jama.267.6.827.

Sloan, F. A., Trogdon, J. G., Curtis, L. H., & Schulman, K. A. (2004). The effect of dementia on outcomes and process of care for Medicare beneficiaries admitted with acute myocardial infarction. *J Am Geriatr Soc, 52*(2), 173-181. doi:10.1111/j.1532-5415.2004.52052.x.

Sullivan-Marx, E. M. (1994). Delirium and physical restraint in the hospitalized elderly. *Image J Nurs Sch, 26*(4), 295-300.

The Hospital Elder Life Program. (2003). Gerontology News. *The Gerontological Society of America, 2.*

Wanich, C. K., Sullivan-Marx, E. M., Gottlieb, G. L., & Johnson, J. C. (1992). Functional status outcomes of a nursing intervention in hospitalized elderly. *Image J Nurs Sch, 24*(3), 201-207.

Wing, R. R., Phelan, S., & Tate, D. (2002). The role of adherence in mediating the relationship between depression and health outcomes. *J Psychosom Res, 53*(4), 877-881. doi:10.1016/S0022-3999(02)00315-X

Young, L. J., & George, J. (2003). Do guidelines improve the process and outcomes of care in delirium? *Age Ageing, 32*(5), 525-528. doi:10.1093/ageing/afg094.

Zarit, S. H., Reever, K. E., & Bach-Peterson, J. (1980). Relatives of the impaired elderly: Correlates of feelings of burden. *Gerontologist, 20*(6), 649-655.

Zuccala, G., Pedone, C., Cesari, M., Onder, G., Pahor, M., Marzetti, E. et al. (2003). The effects of cognitive impairment on mortality among hospitalized patients with heart failure. *Am J Med, 115*(2), 97-103. doi:10.1016/S0002-9343(03)00264-X.

doi:10.1300/J027v26n04_05

Patterns of Emergency Care Use in Residential Care Settings: Opportunities to Improve Quality of Transitional Care in the Elderly

Pamela Parsons, PhD, RN
Peter A. Boling, MD

SUMMARY. Emergent care is a prominent feature in the complex matrix of care transitions for vulnerable elders. This article evaluates local patterns of emergent care transport using ambulance transport data for the year 2003, analyzed by residential setting (independent senior apartments, licensed residential care and nursing homes). Significant differences were found between categories and between facilities within categories (p < .001). The more than three-fold difference in ambulance transport rate between nursing homes reinforces the need to recognize these transitions as quality indicators. Differences between senior apartments and licensed residential care settings provide initial insight

Pamela Parsons is Assistant Professor, Department of Medicine and Peter A. Boling is Professor, Department of Medicine, both at Virginia Commonwealth University School of Medicine, Richmond, VA.

Address correspondence to: Pamela Parsons, PhD, Department of Medicine, Virginia Commonwealth University, P.O. Box 980102, Richmond, VA 23298 (E-mail: pparsons@vcu.edu).

[Haworth co-indexing entry note]: "Patterns of Emergency Care Use in Residential Care Settings: Opportunities to Improve Quality of Transitional Care in the Elderly." Parsons, Pamela and Peter A. Boling. Co-published simultaneously in *Home Health Care Services Quarterly*® (The Haworth Press, Inc.) Vol. 26, No. 4, 2007, pp. 79-92; and: *Charting a Course for High Quality Care Transitions* (ed: Eric A. Coleman) The Haworth Press, Inc. 2007, pp. 79-92. Single or multiple copies of this article are available for a fee from The Haworth Document Delivery Service [1-800-HAWORTH, 9:00 a.m. - 5:00 p.m. (EST). E-mail address: docdelivery@haworthpress.com].

suggesting opportunities for quality improvement in these community settings. doi:10.1300/J027v26n04_06 *[Article copies available for a fee from The Haworth Document Delivery Service: 1-800-HAWORTH. E-mail address: <docdelivery@haworthpress.com> Website: <http://www.HaworthPress. com> © 2007 by The Haworth Press, Inc. All rights reserved.]*

KEYWORDS. Home care services, care transitions

INTRODUCTION

Care transitions have justly received increasing attention and rate of emergent care use is an important quality indicator. Emergency transport rates for community dwelling elders have been documented as high as 179 per 1,000 persons per year with over 15 million elders using the hospital emergency department (ED) in 1995(Ackermann et al., 1998; Strange, & Chen, 1998; Svenson, 2000). Studies of large data sets have shown that multiple factors correlate with emergent care use, including patient co-morbidity and care processes (Phillips et al., 2005). Several studies have shown that pro-active care management can reduce hospitalization rates, both for particular diagnoses such as congestive heart failure and for a broad spectrum of conditions when they occur in conjunction with co-morbidity and risk factors for frailty (Aminzadeh & Dalziel, 2002; McCusker & Verdon, 2006; Murtaugh & Litke, 2002).

Emergent care use comprises part of the Medicare home health quality program, is a focus in the Quality Improvement Organizations' eighth scope of work (Rollow, Lied & McGann, 2006), and is one of the published characteristics selected for Home Health Care Compare (www. Medicare.gov). Emergent care use is also an ACOVE (Assessing Care of Vulnerable Elders) quality indicator for selected conditions (Shekelle et al., 2001). Curiously, CMS does not use emergent care as a quality measure for nursing homes, though high rates of hospitalization for nursing home residents are well documented (Murtaugh & Litke, 2002; Hutt et al., 2002).

Little is yet known about local patterns of emergent care use and particularly about transfers of vulnerable community-dwelling persons who are defined as individuals at increased risk of death or functional decline (Saliba et al., 2001) between residences and hospital emergency departments (ED). A better understanding of transfers and reasons for costly use of emergent ambulance transport from residential care settings could (a) provide insights into factors that contribute to the transfers; (b) provide opportunity for quality improvement by establishing variation between and within setting type; and (c) a better understanding of the patients that rare transferred may facilitate more effective targeting of programs for quality improvement.

Emergent care rate may be driven by a complex array of factors, including living setting characteristics, process of care (e.g., timely access to needed services and high-quality decision-making by health care providers), and patient acuity. Because emergency transport is a discrete, measurable event, patterns of emergent care transport offer a window on care processes for individuals living in structured group living facilities (nursing home and licensed residential care facilities) or residing independently in congregate housing. Study of transition patterns, including differences in rate between categories of setting and between sites within a category, should be an important step in targeting additional supports and improving care processes.

METHODS

To study patterns of emergent acute care transport in Richmond, Virginia we used ambulance service data. Richmond Ambulance Authority (RAA) has an exclusive contract to provide all emergent ambulance services in Richmond city. If volunteer rescue squads or other organizations provide such transports in Richmond they file reports with RAA where a database contains detailed records including patient identifiers, time, primary complaint, and address of origin and destination. We obtained a file containing all Richmond transports in CY2003 with unique patient identifiers removed. We coded the addresses of all nursing homes, licensed residential homes or domiciliary care settings, congregate apartment buildings, and hospital EDs.

Residences were classified in three categories: independent living apartments, licensed residential care, and nursing home. Independent living apartments were defined as facilities where residents perform all activities of daily living and instrumental activities of daily living without requiring assistance from any staff members. Independent senior housing includes subsidized public housing plus private-pay congregate high-rise apartment complexes.

Licensed residential care was defined as congregate residential settings that provide or coordinate personal and health care services, 24-hour supervision, and assistance for care maintenance for four or more adults who are aged, infirm or disabled. Using the Virginia Uniform Assessment Instrument, residents meet criteria for residential care if they have at least one of the following: (a) dependent in only one of seven activities of daily living (bathing, dressing, toileting, transferring, bowel function, bladder function, and eating/feeding; (b) dependent in one or more of four independent activities of daily living (meal preparation, housekeeping, doing laundry, and money management); (c) dependent in medication administration. Some of the licensed residential care facilities are located in older apartment buildings that vary considerably in the character of the physical plans, size and skills sets of staff. These facilities were omitted if the focus of services was predominantly psychiatric care or care of disabled young adults.

Nursing homes are licensed as such, and defined as any facility where the primary function is provision on a continuing basis of nursing services and health-related services for treatment and inpatient care of two or more non-related individuals (Castle & Sonon, 2006). In Richmond, beds in all three facility types are usually full and many facilities have a waiting list.

Within our proposed framework, facility transport rates were calculated as the number of annual transports, urgent and non-urgent from a given living setting to any destination divided by the number of beds in that living setting, thus providing a fixed denominator (number of beds), while the numerator is not fixed (older adults may move in and out of the facility) for the analysis. Urgent transports were defined as emergency room destinations while non-urgent transports were defined as any alternate destination including, but not limited to physician office, dialysis, and outpatient care settings. We compared patterns of transport both within and across the three categories of living setting. The nursing home analysis was limited to 5 facilities because it was necessary for facilities to be located within Richmond city limits so that RAA would have all emergent transports in their database. Persons less than age 65 were included, as they are a portion of the population within these environments which primarily serve the elderly.

We then conducted a sub-analysis of reason for transport in all nursing home transfers. Each transport is assigned a problem code by the emergency rescue squad (EMS) upon arrival at the nursing home, which is validated in the emergency room where the code may be updated. We cleaned the data and analyzed patterns and similarities. Transport codes were assigned to categories, grouped either by diagnosis or presenting symptom. The problem code "falls," was retained to capture the numbers of these important adverse events requiring emergent medical evaluation.

The code for shortness of breath may subsume either pulmonary (e.g., COPD or pneumonia) or cardiac (e.g., congestive heart failure) etiologies. Cardiac arrest requiring cardiopulmonary resuscitation was left unaltered. The category "diabetic complications" includes both hyper and hypoglycemic episodes, with most involving hypoglycemia. The category "gastrointestinal" includes abdominal pain, gastrointestinal bleeding, and nausea and vomiting. Codes that did not fit any established category were labeled "miscellaneous."

RESULTS

As shown in Table 1, 13 independent living settings, 22 residential homes, and 5 nursing homes generated 3,985 ambulance transports. Bed capacity averaged 178 (range 60-198) for nursing homes; 78 (range 14-175) for residential care; and 191 (range 64-274) for independent settings. Average age of those transported was 70 (range 18-111).

Mean transport rates were highest for nursing homes, intermediate for licensed residential care settings, and lowest for independent living apartment buildings as shown in Table 2. There were highly significant differences in rate between categories and between facilities within each category ($p < 001$). Hierarchical regression showed that both facility type and the identity of the individual facility predicted transport rate ($p < 001$). Building capacity was not independently associated with transport rates.

Lastly, we examined diagnosis and problem codes for transports originating in nursing homes (Table 3).

TABLE 1. Facility Characteristics

Facility type	No. of facilities	Mean bed capacity	Mean age in years	Gender (% female)	Total No. transfers
Independent apartments	13	191 (±64-274) SD 67.340	73.57 (±32-104) SD 16.334	65	1274
Licensed residential care	22	77 (±14-175) SD 38.316	63.50 (± 21-111) SD 17.550	47	1319
Nursing home	5	178 (±60-198) SD 36.314	74.66 (±22-111) SD 15.027	67	1392

TABLE 2. Transport Rates (Transports Per Occupant-Year)

Facility category	No. of facilities	High for category	Low for category	Mean for category (SD)	Individual facility	Crude rate
Independent	13	1.47	0.12	0.79 (0.40)		
Residential	22	2.50	0.16	1.48 (0.58)		
Nursing home (NH)	5	3.40	0.98	2.32 (1.04)	NH A	0.98
					NH B	1.36
					NH C	1.39
					NH D	1.40
					NH E	3.40

TABLE 3. Percent of Patients Transported from Nursing Home by Problem Code

Diagnoses/ Reasons for transport	NH A N = 60	NH B N = 128	NH C N = 196	NH D N = 198	NH E N = 196
Non-Urgent	34.5	4.6	22.4	5.6	33.5
Miscellaneous	7.4	15.1	11.9	19.6	13.8
Dyspnea/shortness of breath	9.9	14.3	10.2	11.2	10.1
Cardiac arrest	4.9	0.8	3.4	1.1	0.1
Cardiac arrhythmia	3.7	1.6	3.4	3.6	2.5
Seizure	0	0	3.0	2.9	2.1
Falls	4.9	8.7	6.8	5.1	2.8
Stroke	2.5	0.8	0.4	2.5	0.6
Musculoskeletal pain/injury	7.4	12.7	7.3	8.3	4.0
Unconscious	6.2	7.9	13.2	6.5	6.1
Urinary tract infection	0	2.4	0.4	1.4	1.0
Fever/Sepsis	2.5	4.0	2.6	5.1	4.6
Pneumonia	0	4.8	2.6	0.7	1.0
Psych/Behavioral	2.5	4.8	2.6	6.5	4.8
Diabetic complication	2.5	1.6	2.1	1.1	2.4
Generalized weakness	1.2	4.0	3.4	5.4	3.0
Gastrointestinal	9.9	11.9	4.3	13.4	7.6
*Total = 100%					

N = Beds at facility

DISCUSSION

The most striking observation is the substantial difference in transport rates both between facility types and between facilities within each category. The within-category variation is most marked in the independent and residential categories where the range is more than 10-fold. It is apparent that living location is a proxy for risk of transfer: Since level of care does reflect disease burden, it was no surprise to find a gradient of mean transport rates between categories, rising from independent (0.8) to residential (1.5) settings and 2.4 in nursing homes. Looking within settings however, some senior apartment buildings (1.5) and licensed residential care settings (2.5) had transport rates exceeding those seen in four of the five study nursing homes. Evaluation of demographic, social and cultural aspects within these settings may reveal insight into the marked differences in utilization patterns.

Variation in rates within domicile categories raises interesting questions. To what extent is ED use determined by co-morbidity, rather than care process and access to timely and well-developed medical care systems on-site? Are some variations due largely to physician practice patterns? How much ED use is preventable? Generally, based on studies of small and large area variation (Berwick et al., 2003) experts suggest that improved efficiency (similar or better outcomes at lower cost) can occur using performance improvement and system re-design. There is evidence that changes in staffing, care process, and physician behavior can reduce acute care use (Yaggy et al., 2006; Naylor et al., 2004).

We focused in more detail on the nursing homes in our database. It is known that nursing home residents are frequently transferred to EDs and as many as 40 percent of those transitions result in costly hospital admissions (Ackerman et al., 1998). Our pilot study examined one community and found differences in rate and reason for transition by setting. One nursing home (E) stood out. Having practiced in all 5 nursing homes, we can appreciate differences in care systems that may contribute to the observed differences in transport rate, and this invites further study. The variation in transition rates lends credence to tracking emergency room use and hospitalization, adjusted for case mix, as quality indicators for nursing homes as is now done for home health agencies.

Studying reasons for transport, we found consistent patterns across nursing homes with higher transport rates for falls, musculoskeletal injuries, and abdominal symptoms. More questions arise: the high rate of falls and musculoskeletal injury raise concern for safety measures and care process. There were also apparent differences between facilities in a few categories, such as rate of non-emergent transport, which was notably higher in facilities A, C, and E. This may result from housing unique sub-populations (example dialysis patients), or employing care processes like using specialized hospital-based wound care centers rather than developing such programs at the nursing home. The relatively large proportion of residents that were transported unconscious broaches concern for delay in assessment and treatment, and nursing home E (highest overall transfer rate) had a somewhat higher proportion of transports in this diagnostic category. Most nursing home residents develop warning signs before reaching a state of unresponsiveness from dehydration or sepsis, which are often diagnosed once unresponsive nursing home patients are evaluated.

Within independent living settings, we know less about functional performance, health of residents, or use of health services, in part because these settings are protected by the privacy act of the Housing Authority. Yet, residents in these sites are vulnerable. Most are declining in health and social supports and have moved to obtain financial aid and services such as housekeeping, laundry, food services, checking services, and sometimes personal care. What data we have indicate that those who live in residential care facilities are more frail, disabled and medically ill than average community dwelling elders, require additional supports and lack access to care services (Yaggy et al., 2006; Ball et al., 2004)

When examining these transition patterns, with emphasis on the high rate of transport, it is important to include the possible impact of current regulatory standards and oversight that may impact reasons for transport. These regulatory standards, which affect each individual setting type within a health system policy "silo," additively result in findings such as we have discovered. For example, Joint Commission on Accreditation of Health Care Organization standards (2001) address discharge planning care coordination from the hospital perspective, requiring only evidence of care coordination among health care professions and services directly delivered within the site of the provision of care, but do not necessitate care coordination across sites. From the community perspective, the Outcome and Assessment Information Set (OASIS) for home health patients, also does not address the exchange of information across settings, with no quality measure that actually helps assure that this process takes place. Readmission to acute care is captured within OASIS as an indicator for poor quality, but there remains no targeted standard to capture the exchange of information related to transitions, which is the key process that may help reduce these readmissions. This lack of standardization in the way care is delivered across settings easily leads to fragmented care, with complex chronically ill residents returning to community settings at high risk for transition errors and clinical instability. This discontinuity coupled with lack of clinical and social support ultimately results in return to acute care settings.

Within the nursing home setting, heavy federal regulatory oversight and intense state survey inspections lead to fear of litigation, often forming the impetus for nursing administration's and medical provider decisions for frequent transition to acute care. Also, holding to the concept of the "silo effect" the federally mandated data reporting system within the nursing home setting captures extensive data on patient status and staffing, but does not designate any standard related to transition process across settings, including a striking lack of requirement of reporting emergency room visits.

Lastly financial incentives may influence transport patterns, particularly from the nursing home setting. It was originally surmised that the change to a Prospective Payment System (PPS) by the Centers for Medicare and Medicaid Services (CMS) for Medicare (Part A) skilled nursing facility (SNF) care might adversely affect the quality of care, however recent evaluations have shown no effect on hospitalization or transfers to acute care for the residents that receive these skilled services, thus supporting the efficiency of this capitated system (Wodchis, Frieds & Hirth, 2004). Other financially driven strategies to control transition patterns and acute care utilization include structured models. Evercare (a managed care program using nursing parishioners to provide nursing home care) has positively affected acute care utilization for nursing home residents through case-management. Programs for All Inclusive Care for the Elderly (PACE), have developed efficient systems to provide care across the continuum for community dwelling elders whereas other community such as the have shown little effect on acute care transfer rates, but have reduced long-term nursing home use (Friedman, 2005; Kane et al., 2004). Each of these methods provides examples of managed care attempts to address transition issues with case-management while conserving costs. Generally, evidence based evaluation supports managed care programs with comprehensive geriatric care as an effective means to reduce acute care utilization as compared to Medicare fee-for-service. Within our local setting, in Richmond Virginia, programs of structured managed care for the elderly are not currently in place, and Medicare fee-for-service may be a driver for decisions to transition within all types of facility settings (Lin et al., 2006).

The need to know more is pressing. Our society is creating a diverse spectrum of community housing options for the growing elderly population, many of whom are aging in place with medical co-morbidity and frailty. Nursing homes, assisted living, and independent living settings increasingly overlap when it comes to housing frail and vulnerable sub-populations. Beside the cost, using emergent care often causes individuals to be forced into a new living situation, disrupting not only chronic health care, but also the individual's social life. In many residences, medical care delivery and service models are poorly developed or are not known. As we proceed, we must also acknowledge a tension between the need for affordable housing options like assisted living, senior apartments, and the more organic Naturally Occurring Retirement Communities (NORCs) (Massotti et al., 2006), the need to control health care costs, and the risk of "medicalizing" these environments which can change their culture and raise the specter of increasing regulatory oversight.

If our observations are confirmed, and the large observed differences in transport rates are not entirely due to pre-existing medical co-morbidity, we can speculate about service planning to improve outcomes. Targeted comprehensive geriatric assessment for at-risk community-dwelling elders may save lives and reduce nursing home use (Stuck et al., 2002) Screening interventions could address problems like the highly prevalent yet unrecognized vitamin D deficiency recently documented in several studies (Becker, 2003 & Leslie & Roe, 2003); this condition has been associated with both fall risk and fractures. Medication errors offer other opportunities (Frey & Rahman, 2003).

To systematically improve care processes and outcomes, we need a multi-faceted delivery model that is patient-centered and provides timely access to care. A key component is home health care plus mobile medical care, which can reduce dependence on institutional acute care in these less "medical" living settings. Residents of independent senior housing and licensed residential care are eligible for Medicare home health services as long as they meet homebound and skilled care criteria. Agencies in turn can reduce hospitalization rates using quality improvement methods (Shaughnessy et al., 2002). Mobile medical care models are emerging that have also been reported to improve satisfaction and reduce costs.

One potential risk of strategies designed to manage patient problems in their primary domicile is delaying needed hospital care and causing needless deaths or other adverse outcome. There is evidence that better outcomes can be achieved safely; models of care in nursing homes, some involving advance practice nurses, have produced lower hospitalization rates without increased mortality or decline in other quality measures (Kane et al., 2004; Berwick et al., 2003).

Finally, experts have recently proposed a separate research agenda focused on transitional care. It is a multifaceted, complex entity and requires systematic evaluation within multiple domains. Successful evaluation entails examining patterns of transition and the medical etiologies associated with these events. However, to foster evidence-based decision-making that optimizes patient movement during an episode of care, we must include the trajectory of the process, organizational variables, socioeconomic and cultural factors surrounding transitions, as well as health care costs (Boockvar & Vladeck, 2004). CMS has recently been charged with this focus (Policy Council Document, Post-Acute Care Reform, 2006). Our findings support the need to better define this matrix. In nursing home and residential care settings, appropriate action steps to improve the overuse and misuse of health care system resources related to transitions involve system-level performance measurement and evaluation. Process measures should include transfer of needed information and whether pre and post transition care measures are correctly instituted (Colman & Berenson, 2004).

LIMITATIONS

This is a preliminary study. It depends on the validity of ambulance data, and does not include care setting characteristics or important patient characteristics such as functional status, presence of DNR orders, and various co-morbidities. Linking patient-specific data with the entire transition process, including home health agency and hospital data, primary care utilization information, facility-specific care systems, sociocultural variables, and costs would provide additional insight.

CONCLUSION

This preliminary study describes patterns of acute care service use by living site in Richmond, Virginia. The marked variation in emergency transport rate within a given facility type suggests that care process or resident characteristics may differ between sites, and the size of the differences suggests potential issues with care quality. Transport rate also varies between setting types with nursing homes demonstrating higher rates than residential care and senior apartments. The significance of our initial findings is the implication that high transfer rates within setting type may indicate a need for standardization regarding transfer processes from one setting to the next, and increased utilization of outpatient linking services, such as home health. Our next step is to further analyze transport patterns and combine ambulance data with patient-level data, setting-specific data and other measures of utilization.

REFERENCES

Ackerman, RJ, Kemle, KA, Voget, RL, Griffin, & RC, Jr. (1998). Emergency department use by nursing home residents. *Annals of Emergency Medicine*, 31, 749-757.

Aminzadeh, F, & Dalziel, WB. (2002). Older adults in the emergency department: A systematic review of patterns of use, adverse outcomes, and effectiveness of interventions. *Annals of Emergency Medicine*, 39, 238-247.

Ball, MM, Perkins, MM. Whittington, FJ, Connell, BR, Hollingsworth, C, King, SV, Elrod, CL & Combs, BL. (2004). Managing decline in assisted living: the key to aging in place. *Journal of Gerontology, B Psychological Science and Sociological Science*, 59, S202-S212.

Becker, C. (2003). Clinical evaluation for osteoporosis. (2003). *Clinics in Geriatric Medicine*, 19, 299-320.

Berwick, DM, DeParles, NA, Eddy DM , Ellwood, PM, Enthoven, AC, Halvorson, GC, Kizer, KW et al. (2003). Paying for performance: Medicare should lead. *Health Affairs (Millwood)*, 22, 8-10.

Boockvar, K, & Vladeck BC. (2004). Improving the quality of transitional care for persons with complex care needs. *Journal of the American Geriatrics Society,* 52, 855-856.

Castle, N, & Sonon K. (2006).Internet resources and searching for a residential care facility: What information is available for consumers? *The Journal of Applied Gerontology*, 25, 214-233.

Coleman, EA, & Berenson, RA. (2004). Lost in transition: Challenges and opportunities for improving the quality of transitional care. *Annals of Internal Medicine*, 141, 533-536.

Frey, D & Rahman, A. (2003). Medication management: An evidence-base model that decreases adverse events *Home Healthcare Nurse,* 21, 404-41.

Friedman, SM, Stenwachs, DM, Rathouz, PJ, Burton, LC, & Mukamel, D. (2005). Characteristics predicting nursing home admission in the Program of All- Inclusive Care for Elderly people. *Gerontolologist*, 45(2), 157-166.

Hutt, E, Ecord, M, Eilersten, TB, Frederickson, E, & Kramer, AM. (2002). Precipitants of emergency room visits and acute hospitalization in short-stay Medicare nursing home residents. *Journal of the American Geriatrics Society*, 50, 223-229.

Joint Commission on Accreditation of Healthcare Organizations. 2001 Standards and Intent Statements-Section 1: Patient Focused Functions. Hospital Accrediation

Standards 2001. Oakbrook Terrace: *Joint Commission on Accreditation of Health-Care Organizations*, 69-156.

Kane, RL, Flod, S, Bershadsky, B, & Keckhafer, G. (2004). Effect of an innovative Medicare managed care program on the quality of care for nursing home residents *Gerontologist*, 44, 94-193.

Lin, WC, Kan, RL, Mehr, DR, Madsen, RW, & Petroski, GF. (2006). Changes in the use of postacute care during the initial Medicare payment reforms. *Health Services Research*, 41(4 pt 1), 1338-1356.

Leslie, WD & Rose, EB. (2003). Preventing falls in elderly persons. *New England Journal of Medicine*, 348:1816-1818.

Masotti, PJ, Fick, R, Johnson-Masotti, A, & MacLeod S. (2006). *American Journal of Public Health*, 96, 1164-1170.

McCusker, J. & Verdon, J. (2006). Do geriatric interventions reduce emergency department visits? A systematic review. *Journal of Gerontology, A Biological Science and Medical Science*, 61, 53-62.

Murtaugh, CM & Litke, A. (2002). Transitions through postacute and long-term care settings: Patterns of use and outcomes for a national cohort of elders. *Medical Care*, 40, 227-236.

Naylor, MD, Brooten, DA, Campbell, RL, Maislin, G, McCauley, KM, & Schwartzk JS. (2004). Transitional care of older adults hospitalized with heart failure: A randomized, controlled trial. *Journal of the American Geriatrics Society, 52*, 675-684.

Newcomer, R, Kang, T & Graham, C. (2006). Outcomes in nursing home transition case-management program targeting new admissions. *Gerontologist*, 46(3), 385-390.

Phillips, CD, Holan,S, Sherman, M, Spector, W, & Hawes, C. (2005). Medicare expenditures for residents in assisted living: Data from a national study. Health Services Research, Residents in assisted living: data from a national study. *Health Services Research*, 40, 373-388

Phillips, VL, Paul, W, Becker, FR, Osterweil, D, Ouslander, JG (2000). Health care utilization by old-old long-term care facility residents: How do Medicare fee-for-service and capitation rates compare? *Journal of the American Geriatrics Society*, 48(10), 1330-1336.

Policy Council Document, Post-Acute Care Reform Plan, September 28,2006. http://www.cms.hhs.gov/QualityInititaivesGenInfo/dlowloads/QualityPACFullReport.pdf

Rollow, W, Lied TR, McGann P, Poyer, J, LaVoie, L, Kambic, RT, Bratzler, DW et al. (2006). Assessment of the Medicare quality improvement organization program. *Annals of Internal Medicine*, 145, 343-346.

Saliba, D, Elliott, M, Rubenstein, LZ, Solomon, DH, Young, RT, Kamberg, CJ, Roth, C, Maclean, CH, Shekelle, PG, SLoss EM & Wenger, NS. (20001), The Vulnerable Elders Survey: A tool for identifying vulnerable older people in the community, *Journal of the American Geriatrics Society*, 49(12), 1691-1699.

Shekelle PG, MacLean, CH, Morton, SC, & Wenger, NS (2001). ACOVE quality indicators, *Annals of Internal Medicine*, 135, 653-667.

Shaughnessy, PW, Hittle, DF, Crisler, KS, Powell, MC, Richard AA, Kramers, AM, Schlenker, RE et al. (2002). Improving patient outcomes of home health care: Findings from two demonstration trials of outcome-based quality improvement. *Journal of the American Geriatrics Society*, 50, 1354-1364.

Strange, GR, & Chen, EH (1998). Use of emergency departments by elder patients: A five-year follow-up study. *Academy of Emergency Medicine*, 31, 749-757.

Stuck, AE, Egger, M, Hammer, A, Minder CE, & Beck, JC (2002). Home visits to prevent nursing home admission and functional decline in elderly people: A systemic review and meta-regression analysis *Journal of the American Medical Association*, 287, 1022-1028.

Svenson, JE. (2000). Patterns of use of emergency medical transport: A population-based study, *American Journal of Emergency Medicine*, 18, 130-134.

Wodehis, W, Frieds, B, & Hirth, R. (2004). The effect of Medicare's prospsective payment system on discharge outcomes of skilled nursing facility residents. *Inquiry*, 41, 418-434.

Yaggy, SD, Michener, JL, Yaggy, D, Champagne, MT, Silberberg, M, Ly, M, Johnson, F, & Yarnall, KS (2006). Just for us: An academic medical center-community partnership to maintain the health of a frail low-income senior population. *Gerontologist*, 46, 271-276.

doi:10.1300/J027v26n04_06

The Central Role of Performance Measurement in Improving the Quality of Transitional Care

Eric A. Coleman, MD, MPH
Carla Parry, PhD, MSW, MA
Sandra A. Chalmers, MPH
Amita Chugh, BS
Eldon Mahoney, PhD

SUMMARY. The objectives of this study were: (1) to demonstrate the ability of the Care Transitions Measure (CTM) to identify care deficiencies; (2) to devise and implement a quality improvement approach designed to remedy these deficiencies; (3) to assess the impact of the quality improvement approach on CTM scores; and (4) to test whether the CTM-3 predicts return to the emergency department. The CTM was found to be a sensitive tool able to capture changes in performance. The 3-item CTM was found to significantly predict post-hospital return to the emergency department within the first 30 days ($p = 0.004$). doi:10.1300/J027v26n04_07

Eric A. Coleman, Carla Parry, Sandra A. Chalmers and Amita Chugh are all affiliated with Care Transitions Program, Division of Health Care Policy and Research, University of Colorado at Denver Health Sciences Center, Denver, CO. Eldon Mahoney is affiliated with PeaceHealth, Bellingham, WA.

Address correspondence to: Eric A. Coleman, Division of Health Care Policy and Research, University of Colorado at Denver Health Sciences Center, 13611 East Colfax Avenue, Suite 100, Aurora CO 80045 (E-mail: Eric.Coleman@uchsc.edu).

This study was supported by a grant from the Commonwealth Fund of New York.

[Haworth co-indexing entry note]: "The Central Role of Performance Measurement in Improving the Quality of Transitional Care." Coleman, Eric A. et al. Co-published simultaneously in *Home Health Care Services Quarterly*® (The Haworth Press, Inc.) Vol. 26, No. 4, 2007, pp. 93-104; and: *Charting a Course for High Quality Care Transitions* (ed: Eric A. Coleman) The Haworth Press, Inc. 2007, pp. 93-104. Single or multiple copies of this article are available for a fee from The Haworth Document Delivery Service [1-800-HAWORTH, 9:00 a.m. - 5:00 p.m. (EST). E-mail address: docdelivery@haworthpress.com].

KEYWORDS. Care transitions, performance measurement, care coordination, quality improvement

INTRODUCTION

Transitional care has been defined as a set of actions designed to ensure the coordination and continuity of care received by patients as they transfer between different locations of care (Coleman & Boult, 2003). Older patients with complex care needs frequently require care from different health care settings. Poor coordination of care during transitions across these settings threatens patient safety, increases cost of care due to recidivism, and can create undue burden not only on the patient but also for family caregivers (Coleman & Berenson, 2004).

The 2005 Institute of Medicine report, "Performance Measurement: Accelerating Improvement," explicitly identified transitional care as one of three priority areas for performance measurement (Committee on Redesigning Health Insurance Performance Measures & Board on Health Care Services, 2006). However, lack of performance measurement in the area of transitional care has presented a significant barrier to improving quality. The Care Transitions Measure (CTM) was developed with substantial input from patients and family caregivers and has been rigorously designed and tested to fill this gap (Coleman et al., 2002; Coleman, Mahoney, & Parry, 2005). The CTM includes 15 items (the CTM-15) (Figure 1).

The CTM assesses the quality of a transition from the perspective of the patient. Because its items are "actionable," it can thus help to guide quality improvement efforts. Responses to the CTM have been shown to predict recidivism to the hospital (Coleman et al., 2005). In an effort to reduce response burden, a 3-item version of the CTM (the CTM-3) was developed, tested, and subsequently endorsed for public reporting by the National Quality Forum in May 2006 (The National Quality Forum, 2006).

The CTM is being applied to a broad range of diseases and populations by the over 1000 groups that have requested permission to use of the

FIGURE 1. The Care Transitions Measure[1,2]

1. Before I left the hospital, the staff and I agreed about clear health goals for me and how these would be reached.
2. The hospital staff took my preferences and those of my family or caregiver into account in deciding what my health care needs would be when I left the hospital.*
3. The hospital staff took my preferences and those of my family or caregiver into account in deciding where my health care needs would be met when I left the hospital.
4. When I left the hospital, I had all the information I needed to be able to take care of myself.
5. When I left the hospital, I clearly understood how to manage my health.
6. When I left the hospital, I clearly understood the warning signs and symptoms I should watch for to monitor my health condition.
7. When I left the hospital, I had a readable and easily understood written plan that described how all of my health care needs were going to be met.
8. When I left the hospital, I had a good understanding of my health condition and what makes it better or worse.
9. When I left the hospital, I had a good understanding of the things I was responsible for in managing my health.*
10. When I left the hospital, I was confident that I knew what to do to manage my health.
11. When I left the hospital, I was confident I could actually do the things I needed to do to take care of my health.
12. When I left the hospital, I had a readable and easily understood written list of the appointments or tests I needed to complete within the next several weeks.
13. When I left the hospital, I clearly understood the purpose for taking each of my medications.*
14. When I left the hospital, I clearly understood how to take each of my medications, including how much I should take and when.
15. When I left the hospital, I clearly understood the possible side effects of each of my medications.

*Indicates CTM-3 Items (items 2, 9, and 13)

[1] © Eric A. Coleman, MD, MPH. The CTM was created for use in the public domain. Individuals or institutions interested in using the CTM may download the instrument at http://www.caretransitions.org. No user fees are required.
[2] Scale 1, strongly disagree; 2, disagree; 3, agree; 4, strongly agree

measure. These include health plans, hospitals, home health agencies, quality improvement organizations, government organizations, researchers, and policymakers. The WHO Regional Office for Europe is sponsoring a hospital quality improvement project that will incorporate the CTM in the indicator set to be used in up to 200 hospitals in 10 countries.

The study reported herein focused on a particularly vulnerable transition–an older patient's discharge from hospital–and the ability of the CTM to improve care during this challenging time period. Discharges from the hospital to home (with or without skilled home health care services) were included. The primary goal of this project was to enable a process whereby a hospital identifies its own particular deficiencies in care transitions, develops quality improvement projects that attempt to remedy these deficiencies, and then assesses the impact of the quality improvement efforts. Accordingly, the study was comprised of four inter-related activities: (1) to demonstrate the ability of the CTM to identify care deficiencies; (2) to devise and implement a quality improvement approach designed to remedy these deficiencies; (3) to assess the impact of the quality improvement approach on CTM scores; and (4) to test whether the CTM-3 predicts return to the emergency department, an important attribute for gaining support from clinicians and senior leadership to endorse the measure's routine use in quality improvement efforts.

METHODS

Setting

The study was conducted in a community-based non-profit hospital located in the Pacific Northwest. The Colorado Multiple Institutional Review Board and the institutional review board for the participating hospital approved the study protocols.

Participants

Two distinct, mutually exclusive samples were recruited using identical enrollment criteria. The purpose of the baseline sample was to identify the hospital's deficiencies in transitional care and aimed to recruit 50 patients to complete the CTM. The purpose of the intervention sample was to assess the impact of the quality improvement approach and aimed to recruit 200 patients to complete the CTM. For the latter sample, a total of 192 patients were recruited during the study period. In each sample, the study population included persons aged 65 and older who had been admitted to the study hospital with a diagnosis of diabetes or congestive heart failure (CHF). These two diseases were selected based on: (1) the high likelihood of requiring follow-up care after hospitalization; (2) the high likelihood of requiring medication adjustment as a result of the hospitalization; and (3) the need for ongoing self-management following hospital discharge. Patients were recruited from three hospital wards: cardiology, general medicine, and medical-surgical. Additional eligibility criteria include that the patient be able to provide informed consent, speak English, be reachable by telephone during the 30-day period following hospital discharge, and not permanently reside in a long-term care facility. Informed consent was obtained from all study participants.

Data Sources

Upon enrollment, participants were asked to provide their age, gender, marital status, and ethnicity. The Deyo-modified version of the Charlson co-morbidity score was calculated on all participants using hospital claims data (Deyo, Cherkin, & Ciol, 1992).

Professional survey researchers telephonically assessed patients' responses to the CTM items. These interviews were administered person-to-person (i.e., without automation) and were conducted between 7 and 21 days after hospital discharge.

Study Design

The primary outcome variable of interest was mean CTM-15 scores. The baseline sample was assessed over a one-month period. The intervention sample was assessed longitudinally on a monthly basis between October 2004 and June 2005.

Statistical Analysis

Linear transformation was performed to convert individual and mean scores to a 0-100 scale. Linear regression was performed to assess the relationship between CTM scores following hospitalization and subsequent use of the emergency department, controlling for other independent variables. Use of the emergency department was the dependent variable. Age, gender, marital status, ethnicity, comorbidity score, admitting diagnosis, patient care unit, and CTM scores comprised the independent variables. Monthly changes in mean CTM-15 scores were assessed using a statistical process control framework. The Levene equality of variance test was used to determine statistical significance. All analyses were conducted for the CTM-15 using SPSS Version 12.0.

RESULTS

Patient Characteristics

Demographics of study participants are provided in Table 1. Overall, the population is characterized by advanced age, largely Caucasian, and a slight majority were men. When examining the admitting diagnosis in the intervention population, 34.9% were categorizes as congestive heart failure (CHF), 47.0% as diabetes and 16.4% had both diagnoses.

TABLE 1. Descriptive Statistics for Demographic Variables

	Baseline Sample (N = 50)		Intervention Sample (N = 192)	
Age	Mean = 77.7 S.D = 7.5		Mean = 76.3 S.D. = 6.8	
Gender				
F	10	20.0%	86	44.8%
M	40	80.0%	101	52.6%
missing	0	0.0%	5	2.6%
Marital Status				
Married	23	46.0%	90	46.9%
Widowed	14	28.0%	52	27.1%
Divorced	3	6.0%	11	5.7%
Single	6	12.0%	17	8.9%
Missing	4	8.0%	1	0.5%
Ethnicity				
Caucasian	49	98.0%	183	95.3%
Hispanic	0	0.0%	2	1.0%
Native American	0	0.0%	1	0.5%
Other	1	2.0%	1	0.5%
Unknown	0	0.0%	1	0.5%
Primary Diagnosis				
CHF	18	36.0%	66	34.4%
CHF, Diabetes	9	18.0%	32	16.7%
Diabetes	22	44.0%	90	46.9%
Missing	1	2.0%	4	2.1%
Patient Care Unit				
3rd Medical	7	14.0%	39	20.3%
Cardiovascular	43	86.0%	120	62.5%
Medical Care Unit	0	0.0%	29	15.1%
Comorbidity Index				
0	n/a	n/a	23	12.0%
1	n/a	n/a	47	24.5%
2	n/a	n/a	60	31.3%
3	n/a	n/a	18	9.4%
4+	n/a	n/a	15	7.8%

CTM Scores at Baseline

Table 2 illustrates the baseline mean CTM scores at the aggregate and individual levels. The mean (aggregated) CTM-15 score was 70.2 and the mean CTM-3 score was 69.6. These baseline scores suggested that there was room for improvement in multiple areas. These data were presented to hospital leaders to help guide the design of a quality improvement process that they believed was within the control of hospital ward staff and would be potentially sensitive to change over time.

Quality Improvement Intervention

These care deficiencies were translated into the following clinical care goals: (1) attention to how a patient's illness would impact their life upon returning home; (2) helping patients better understand how to take medications and monitor for potential side effects; and (3) the need for a more comprehensive set of written instructions upon discharge.

TABLE 2. Mean CTM Scores by Item

	Baseline Sample (N = 50)		Intervention Sample (N = 192)	
	Mean	S.D.	Mean	S.D
CTM Item 1	3.03	.499	3.08	.561
CTM Item 2	3.08	.547	3.07	.519
CTM Item 3	3.05	.613	3.05	.534
CTM Item 4	3.21	.528	3.14	.543
CTM Item 5	3.15	.489	3.08	.517
CTM Item 6	3.10	.447	3.12	.510
CTM Item 7	2.92	.664	2.93	.625
CTM Item 8	3.11	.509	3.04	.566
CTM Item 9	3.13	.339	3.09	.470
CTM Item 10	3.08	.480	3.07	.519
CTM Item 11	3.13	.339	3.06	.498
CTM Item 12	3.11	.453	3.09	.533
CTM Item 13	3.03	.560	3.08	.572
CTM Item 14	3.08	.433	3.15	.518
CTM Item 15	2.89	.559	2.86	.570

The following interventions were designed to operationalize the clinical care goals. In-services focused on patient-centered care and improved hospital team care was held on the three hospital care units. New patient educational materials were developed to help patients identify warning signs and symptoms that may indicate that their condition is worsening and steps to take if these occur. Individualized congestive heart failure and diabetes self-management training for patients and their caregivers that emphasize the specific skills they will need after discharge. Hospital ward nurses and discharge planners were encouraged to more actively involve patients and caregivers in the development of discharge plans. Once the discharge care plan was developed, it could be prominently featured in a newly developed section of the health care system's electronic medical record so that they will be available across sites following transfer.

Response of CTM Scores to Intervention

As illustrated in Figure 2, while CTM scores increased significantly during the initial implementation of the intervention, the quality gains were counteracted by discrete events that disrupted stability at a system level. Specifically, CTM scores increased with the "roll-out" of the intervention during months of October, November, and December. These improvements demonstrate that CTM scores are responsive to change in care processes. Measuring quality in this area and providing staff with appropriate directions, tools and support can translate into a better transition experience for patients.

However, over the course of the study period, there were two noteworthy negative events that impacted staff performance of the three study hospital wards (Figure 2). The first was a rumor that the hospital was experiencing financial difficulty that occurred in December 2004. Second, there was a change in nurse staffing policy in February 2005 that led to nurses being re-assigned to new hospital wards in accordance with seniority. As a result, long-standing working relationships were disrupted and new relationships had to be established. Immediately following each of these discreet events, CTM scores were observed to decline. In other words, patients detected this disruption and reported more negative transition experiences. Once system stability was restored, improvements in CTM scores followed but were not sustained after external support for the intervention ended.

A statistical process control framework can be used to examine the influence of the care process intervention and the influence of the negative events. In Figure 2, we see that two points were out of the control limits–December 2004 and March 2005. These two values do not simply represent random variation as the points that precede these them suggest a trend of improvement to December 2004 followed by a decline to March 2005. Independent sample t-test comparing December 2004 and March 2005 demonstrate a statistically significant difference (Levene equality of variance test F < 1 so equal variances assumed and t = 2.27, df = 36, p = .029).

CTM-3 Scores Predict Subsequent Emergency Department Use

The relationship between CTM scores and emergency department use is presented in Table 3. Linear regression analyses revealed care transition quality as measured by the CTM-3 significantly predicted

FIGURE 2. Control Chart: Care Transition Measure Score (Linear)

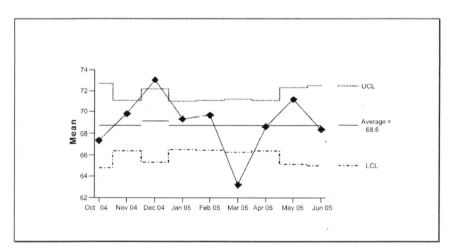

TABLE 3. Relationship Between CTM Scores and Utilization (# ED visits)

	F Statistic	Significance P-value
Model	3.040	.013
Intercept	.166	.685
Co-Morbidity score		
(Deyo)	1.486	.225
Age	.045	.833
CTM Score	4.679	.004

return to the emergency department within 30 days of discharge from the index hospitalization ($p = 0.004$). These analyses were adjusted for age, gender, marital status, ethnicity, hospital ward, admitting diagnosis, and comorbidity score.

DISCUSSION

The findings from this study demonstrate the responsiveness of CTM scores to both positive and negative influences. The CTM scores improved with the roll out of an intervention designed to improve the quality of the transition experience. However, the two negative events counteracted these improvements and illustrate how system level instability is quickly translated from clinical staff to patients. Patients were able to detect how this disruption affected the way they interacted with hospital staff and how this disruption ultimately influenced the quality of their discharge experience. In other words, patients are ideally positioned to judge the quality of the care they receive as they move across settings and the CTM is a sensitive tool specifically designed to capture their experiences. The fact that both CTM-15 scores (previously reported) (Coleman et al., 2005) and CTM-3 scores (reported herein) predict recidivism provides further confirmation for the assertion that the CTM assesses more patient satisfaction. It is indeed, a measure of quality.

Two recent reviews of performance measures that address care coordination and transitional care serves to place the results of this study in context with the literature (Committee on Redesigning Health Insurance Performance Measures et al., 2006; McDonald et al., 2006). Currently, there is a paucity of measures of care coordination or care transitions that are based on patient report. The authors are not aware of any other measures that have been shown to predict important patient outcomes such as recidivism. The findings from this study help diffuse existing controversy over whether patients are able to accurately ascertain the quality of care received with respect to care coordination or transitional care (McDonald et al., 2006). In further support of this position, Nelson and colleagues who have demonstrated that improved scores on hospital discharge planning items translated into financial savings (Nelson & Rust, 1992).

The results of this study are supported by a number of strengths. First, the study was conducted in a community-based hospital, which enhances the generalizability of the findings. Second, the study assessed quality from the perspective of the patients themselves. Third, the study attempted to capture the system-level factors that may have influenced the findings. However, there are several limitations to consider. The study population was predominantly Caucasian and the generalizability to more diverse populations is unknown. The hospital leaders were very motivated to improve care coordination and this may also not be representative of hospitals across the country that may have different priorities. Finally, although the study team attempted to ascertain factors that may have influenced patient responses to the CTM, there may have been undetected factors that may have the influenced findings.

Important implications follow the results of this study. First and foremost, because patients are often the only common thread weaving across various health care settings, they are uniquely positioned to assess the quality of care transitions. The findings from this study strongly suggest that patients are able perceptive to changes in the delivery system that influence their care experience and can reliably judge the quality of their care. The Care Transitions Measure was found to be acceptable to patients in the study and was sensitive to detecting meaningful change in health system performance. Further, the fact that CTM-3 scores predict recidivism firmly establishes this measure as a valuable quality assessment tool rather than simply a satisfaction survey.

The study hospital put forth considerable resources to improving care coordination and initially these efforts appeared to pay dividends. Despite these initial improvements, the positive results were quickly counteracted by external influences as well as by the conclusion of the study. Clearly give the challenges presented by coordinating care across settings, constant vigilance is needed to produce sustained results. Further, coordination of care is particularly vulnerable to system instability and when hospital staff become particularly stressed, attention to discharge preparation may be viewed as more of a discretionary rather than essential task.

Although this study was conducted in a hospital setting, the Care Transitions Measure has been used widely across a broad array of care transfers. Thus the findings from this study have implications for consideration in settings such as skilled nursing facilities and home health care. With respect to the latter, given the national goals for reducing hospital admission (or readmission) among the home health care population (Centers for Medicare and Medicaid Services, 2006), the CTM may prove to be a valuable tool for performance measurement. In this context, home care agencies may choose to use the CTM to assess the short- and long-term impact of their efforts and potentially modify their interventions based on how their clients quality ratings.

In conclusion, the CTM is an important tool for assessing performance in an area that has historically received inadequate attention–transitional care. The CTM is truly patient centered, well accepted by patients, sensitive to meaningful change, and relatively brief. The finding that CTM-3 scores predict recidivism further enhances the value of this tool and its utility for quality improvement efforts.

REFERENCES

Centers for Medicare and Medicaid Services (2006). *Home health quality initiatives: Overview* (http://www.cms.hhs.gov/HomeHealthQualityInits/accessed 2/23/07).

Coleman, E. A. & Berenson, R. A. (2004). Lost in transition: Challenges and opportunities for improving the quality of transitional care. *Ann Intern Med, 141,* 533-536.

Coleman, E. A., & Boult, C., on behalf of the American Geriatrics Society Health Care Systems Committee (2003). Improving the quality of transitional care for persons with complex care needs. *J Am Geriatr Soc, 51,* 556-557.

Coleman, E. A., Eilertsen, T. B., Smith, J. D., Frank, J., Thiare, J. N., Ward, A. et al. (2002). Development and testing of a measure designed to assess the quality of care transitions. *Int J Integrated Care [Access* www.ijic.org], *vol 2.*

Coleman, E. A., Mahoney, E., & Parry, C. (2005). Assessing the quality of preparation for posthospital care from the patient's perspective: the Care Transitions Measure. *Med Care, 43,* 246-255.

Committee on Redesigning Health Insurance Performance Measures, P. a. P. I. P. & Board on Health Care Services (2006). *Performance measurement: accelerating improvement.* Washington DC: Institute of Medicine of the National Academies.

Deyo, R., Cherkin, D., & Ciol, M. (1992). Adapting a clinical morbidity index for use with ICD-9-CM administrative databases. *J Clin Epidemiol, 45,* 613-619.

McDonald, K. M., Sundaram, V., Bravata, D. M., Lewis, R., Lin, N., Paguntalan, H. et al. (2006). Volume 6: Care coordination. In K.G.Shojania, K. M. McDonald, R. M. Wachter, & D. K. Owens (Eds.), *Closing the quality gap: A critical analysis of quality improvement strategies: technical review 9e* (pp. 1-118). Stanford University-UCSF Evidence-based Practice Center, Stanford,CA for Agency for Healthcare Research and Quality Contract No. 290-02-0017.

Nelson, E. C. & Rust, R. T. (1992). Do patient perceptions of quality relate to hospital financial performance? *Journal of Health Care Marketing, 12,* 6-13.

The National Quality Forum (2006). *National voluntary consensus standards for hospital care: Additional priority areas–2005-2006* (http://www.qualityforum.org/docs/hosp_measures/webtx3Hosppublic07-07-06.pdf Accessed 08/22/06). Washington D.C..

doi:10.1300/J027v26n04_07

ReACH National Demonstration Collaborative: Early Results of Implementation

Patricia Simino Boyce, RN, MA, PhD
Penny Hollander Feldman, PhD

SUMMARY. The Reducing Acute Care Hospitalization (ReACH) National Demonstration Collaborative is a two-year multi-wave initiative using a "virtual" Collaborative Learning Model to reduce acute care hospitalization rates among home care patients. ReACH aims to reduce hospitalization to 23%, as recommended by the Centers for Medicare and Medicaid Services in its 8th Scope of Work for Quality Improvement Organizations. This article reports on the early implementation experience of a sample of 17 of 65 home health agencies participating in

Patricia Simino Boyce is Director of the Partnership for Achieving Quality Homecare (PAQH) and the Effort for Quality Improvement and Performance in Home Health Care (EQUIP) at the Visiting Nurse Service of New York. Penny Hollander Feldman is Vice President, Visiting Nurse Service of New York and Director, VNSNY Center for Home Care Policy and Research.

Address correspondence to: Penny H. Feldman, PhD, VNSNY Center for Home Care Policy and Research, 107 E. 70th Street, New York, NY 10021 (E-mail: pfeldman@vnsny.org).

The authors wish to thank Danylle Rudin for her assistance in preparing this article.

This work was supported by the Agency for Healthcare Research and Quality, Grant Number: 5 U18 HS013694-04 and by the Robert Wood Johnson Foundation, Grant No. 042588.

[Haworth co-indexing entry note]: "ReACH National Demonstration Collaborative: Early Results of Implementation." Boyce, Patricia Simino and Penny Hollander Feldman. Co-published simultaneously in *Home Health Care Services Quarterly*® (The Haworth Press, Inc.) Vol. 26, No. 4, 2007, pp. 105-120; and: *Charting a Course for High Quality Care Transitions* (ed: Eric A. Coleman) The Haworth Press, Inc. 2007, pp. 105-120. Single or multiple copies of this article are available for a fee from The Haworth Document Delivery Service [1-800-HAWORTH, 9:00 a.m. - 5:00 p.m. (EST). E-mail address: docdelivery@haworth press.com].

Wave I of ReACH. It examines agency challenges in implementing a structured practice improvement initiative, improving hospital to home transitions and focusing appropriate resources on high risk patients. Lessons learned will inform future home health care quality improvement initiatives. doi:10.1300/J027v26n04_08 *[Article copies available for a fee from The Haworth Document Delivery Service: 1-800-HAWORTH. E-mail address: <docdelivery@haworthpress.com> Website: <http://www.Haworth Press.com> © 2007 by The Haworth Press, Inc. All rights reserved.]*

KEYWORDS. Hospitalization, transitions, home care, quality improvement, practice change, learning collaborative

INTRODUCTION

Evidence suggests that closing the gap between science and practice can reduce acute care hospitalization rates among home care patients (Coleman, Parry, Chalmers, & Sung-Joon,. 2006; Mistiaen & Poote, 2006; Naylor, 2002, 2006; Naylor et al., 1999; Naylor et al., 2004; Phillips et al., 2004; World Health Organization, 2005). Significant variability in rates of hospitalization exists across home care agencies, ranging from 17% to 47% in one study (Delmarva Foundation for Medical Care, 2005). This studye same study found that a risk-adjusted hospitalization rate of 23.16% or less had been attained by 25% (1,787) of all home health agencies. Although the optimal rate of hospitalization is unknown, a panel of home care experts convened in June 2005 to examine available data concluded that there is an opportunity for improvement as evidenced by the variability in rates, and that home health agencies, although not the entire "solution," could help reduce avoidable hospitalizations through practice improvements (K. Pace, personal communication, November 30, 2006).

The Reducing Acute Care Hospitalization (ReACH) National Demonstration Collaborative is a two-year multi-wave initiative using a "virtual" Collaborative Learning Model to reduce acute care hospitalization among home care patients. With support from the national ReACH staff and technical assistance from 16 Quality Improvement Organizations (QIOs) throughout the country, 177 home health agencies are implementing targeted improvement strategies to reduce hospitalization rates among their patients. Participating agencies were recruited directly by their QIOs, who were encouraged to focus on those agencies that had both a high ACH rate and an interest in participating in the ReACH Collaborative.

Through a combination of virtual and face-to-face communications, ReACH provides participating agencies access to breakthrough improvement methods, training and technical assistance to implement effective strategies in everyday practice. Key components of ReACH are:

1. A National Learning Community that includes monthly conference calls, WebEx learning sessions and access to a ListServ and Website
2. Local improvement assistance by the respective QIOs under whose jurisdiction the home health agencies fall, including meetings, conference calls, site visits and technical assistance to individual agencies
3. Regional face to face meetings hosted by the QIOs that provide the opportunity for group discussions, exchange of information and collaborative learning among home health agencies
4. Targeted improvement strategies (e.g., risk-assessment tools and recommended practice changes)
5. Standardized measures capturing processes and outcomes for reducing acute care hospitalizations
6. A web-based data collection and performance tracking system that allows each agency to enter monthly data on specific measures and monitor progress in implementing change strategies and achieving desired outcomes

Recognizing that many agencies will require long term efforts to overcome complex systems problems that contribute to high hospitalization rates, the ReACH Collaborative nevertheless chose to work toward the ambitious goal established by the Centers for Medicare and Medicaid Services (CMS) in its 8th scope of work–a recommended hospitalization rate of 23% for all participating home health agencies by August 2007. To accomplish this, ReACH charges participating agencies with the tasks of:

1. Instituting a quality improvement process to reduce acute care hospitalizations for patients at risk
2. Establishing explicit criteria for admitting patients from hospital and improving their transition to home care
3. Increasing capacity to appropriately screen and intervene for patients at risk of hospitalization
4. Implementing targeted strategies and systems to support effective care management
5. Enhancing communication and coordination with primary care physicians and specialists

This article reports on the early implementation experience of a sample of 17 home care agencies participating in WAVE I of ReACH. In particular, it examines the challenges they faced in implementing a structured practice improvement initiative and adopting a systematic method to identify patients at risk of hospitalization early in their home care stay. The transition into home care–especially the process by which patients are referred from the hospital–is often hurried, and the information available upon home care admission is often conflicting or incomplete. Risk identification, then, can be seen as compensating for transition "failures" that may occur during the patient's journey to home care. Systematic identification and effective management of high-risk patients has been shown to reduce rehospitalization (Naylor, 2002, 2006; Naylor et al., 1999; Naylor et al., 2004) and is important so that home health agencies can target precious clinical resources.

METHODS

Seventeen of the 65 home health agencies participating in Wave I of ReACH were randomly selected to participate in a half hour phone interview that took place approximately four months after the start of the Collaborative. The sample ranged from small, freestanding agencies to very large, network-based and hospital-affiliated agencies. These agencies had a range of 2-6 staff working on the ReACH Collaborative, and three of those sampled had agency leadership participating as active team members. The seventeen agencies represented eleven states and all ten QIOs that participated in Wave I.

The purpose of the interviews was to discuss the materials and support the agency received from ReACH and to solicit input to improve ReACH technical assistance and materials in the future. All 17 agencies agreed to participate. A member of the ReACH project team scheduled and conducted the interviews within a two-week period in July 2006. One person from each agency's team was contacted and an interview scheduled. The purpose of the interview was explained; respondents were assured that their answers would be confidential and that any reports or published results would be presented in aggregate form. Research questions assessed respondents' perceptions of the Collaborative Learning Model, ReACH intervention strategies, home health agencies' selection and testing of of interventions, and respondents' appraisals of the support their agencies received from the ReACH Team and local QIO. (Interview protocol available upon request.) Numeric scores were calculated for all objective questions. In addition, two members of the research team reviewed the qualitative notes from the calls to extract common themes.

Four of the 17 agencies were selected for a second interview to elucidate factors associated with successful reductions in acute care hospitalization. As of July 2006, when selection was made, the four agencies selected had achieved the most significant reductions in their agency-wide hospitalization rate relative to their baseline data. In these interviews, which were about ten minutes long, agencies answered a series of open-ended questions about the structure of their ReACH Collaborative, staff "buy-in," most effective implementation strategies, leadership involvement, and QIO contributions toward the agency's success. Two members of the research team reviewed the notes from these calls to identify crosscutting themes.

RESULTS

Fourteen respondents were active ReACH team members in their home health agencies; eleven also identified themselves as Quality Improvement Specialists. Others were leadership staff or project liaisons representing the ReACH team within their agencies. Baseline acute care hospitalization (ACH) rates ranged from 14% to 68.5%, with an average rate of 26.4%, excluding the 68.5% outlier. Figure 1 presents the distribution of baseline hospitalization rates among the 17 sampled agencies.

Implementation Challenges

The first section of the interview focused on agencies' overall participation in the ReACH Collaborative, particularly on implementation challenges. Of the 17 respondents, 12 reported their agency's participation in the ReACH Collaborative was "somewhat smooth," 4 reported it was "very smooth" and one that it was "not at all smooth." Obtaining adequate, appropriate, committed staff was the most frequently cited implementation challenge, followed by finding time to devote to the project. Some agencies found it difficult to understand the data requirements of the Collaborative, and others found it difficult to integrate the project with larger changes occurring in their organizations (e.g., transition to

FIGURE 1. ACH Baseline Rate for Agencies Completing a ReACH Interview (N = 17)

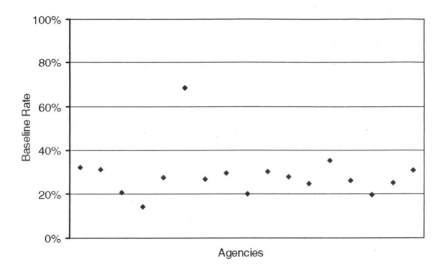

new electronic data systems). Summarized below are the responses to a list of challenges from which respondents could select multiple items:

- Availability of Agency Resources (6 respondents): This included staff shortages and/or challenges in obtaining staff participation and "buy-in." Smaller agencies, in particular, reported that they did not have sufficient resources to adequately focus on the project. Competing priorities were an issue for several agencies.
- Time to Devote to Project (5 respondents): Some respondents indicated that the project was extremely time consuming, including monthly data collection and input as well as planning and implementing change strategies.
- Other (4 respondents): Several agencies were in the process of or had just changed from a paper system to an electronic data system, and assimilating the Collaborative's improvement methods was difficult to do during the agency's technology transition process. Some also found it difficult to locate culturally and linguistically appropriate tools and patient education materials.
- Data Management (3 respondents): A few agencies had difficulty understanding the Collaborative's data collection process. This included instructions for baseline data collection, as well as for monthly tracking of measures.

Agencies addressed these challenges in multiple ways. They worked to integrate the ReACH project into existing initiatives, provide additional staff support to the ReACH team, coordinate ReACH training with existing training schedules and prioritize tasks to maximize available staff time and resources. Many agencies relied heavily on the materials provided by the national ReACH staff to structure and focus their work, and many called on their QIOs for further assistance. A number of agencies had already begun work on acute care hospitalization, which facilitated implementation of the ReACH strategies. In general, securing leadership support was perceived as key, as was investing time up front to engage staff and impress upon them the importance for their patients and their agency of reducing avoidable hospitalizations.

Overall, when asked what was most helpful in facilitating their participation in ReACH, the most commonly cited responses were:

- ReACH resources (13 respondents)
- Prior experience addressing acute care hospitalization issues (12 respondents)
- Committed leadership (12 respondents)
- Support and encouragement from the QIO (11 respondents)
- Staff understanding and acceptance of the need to reduce the agency's acute care hospitalization rate (11 respondents)

At the time of the interviews most agencies were still deeply involved in addressing implementation challenges. Among those prepared to make an initial judgment, the majority viewed their efforts as "somewhat" successful to date.

Identifying Patients at Risk For Hospitalization

A key improvement strategy emphasized by the national ReACH Collaborative staff as the first step in tackling the hospitalization problem was the adoption of a systematic method for identifying patients at high risk of hospitalization. To that end, the Collaborative provided a sample risk assessment tool (available upon request) developed by the Carolinas Center for Medical Excellence based on research in the field (Rosati, Huang, Navaie-Waliser, & Feldman, 2003). Also provided were a set of instructions and a template that agencies could use to test and modify the tool based on the case mix of their particular agency. (Agency-specific case mix data were provided by the QIOs.) The national Collaborative staff also provided information on "rapid cycle" tests of change and encouraged participating agencies to engage in them and to assess their results before adopting any "final" tool or strategy.

When asked to describe their first test of change, all of the respondents described their experience in testing a risk assessment tool and modifying it to address their agency's needs. All of the agencies started out with the materials provided by ReACH, and a half dozen supplemented these with internal reports, chart audits and software applications to identify additional risk factors. Fifteen of the 17 relied on their QIO for assistance in the process, and a half dozen required a great deal of assistance. Following the instructions provided in the ReACH template, most assessed the applicability of the tool to their own agency by selecting random samples of admitted patients who were subsequently hospitalized or not hospitalized and comparing the risk profiles and risk scores of the two groups. Based on the results, most agencies made some adjustments. Some had to repeat this process multiple times in order to get a tool that in their judgment accurately reflected risk in their patient population. A few noted that it had been difficult to narrow organizational factors and patient population characteristics to a limited set of "high risk" factors; it had been surprising to learn what factors were objectively associated with hospitalization risk.

Once a tool had been decided upon, several agencies found that not all of their nurses were using it and made additional modifications to make it more user-friendly. Before widespread implementation, some agencies tested the tool on a small scale: a select group of nurses, one county, or a certain number of patients. Most used logs, Excel spreadsheets or retroactive chart reviews to monitor change. With effectively sequenced tests of change, most agencies settled on a risk assessment tool that was relatively easy for their clinicians to use, although several reported difficulty in testing and implementation. QIO assistance was particularly important to this latter group.

By the end of the four-month period, all 17 agencies had adopted a risk assessment tool. Moreover, all but one of the respondents said that after the ReACH Initiative concluded, their agencies would continue to use these tools and resources when identifying patients at-risk. The remaining agency already required nurses to fill out a risk-assessment tool and would continue to do so. Figure 2 portrays the change in use of a risk assessment tool from baseline through July 2006 for all agencies in the Collaborative. The significant improvement achieved among all 65 Wave I participants indicates that the experience of the 17 agencies represented in the interviews was not atypical.

FIGURE 2. Percentage of Completed Risk Assessments for Wave 1 Agencies (N = 65)

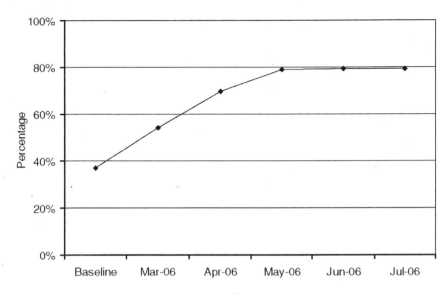

Testing Improvement Strategies

At the time of the interviews, several of the 17 agencies were still in the process of implementing their risk assessment tool and had not started planning for another test of change. Others had already tested additional strategies or were planning to test changes such as "front loading" visits to high risk patients (i.e., providing a higher than average number of visits or contacts in the first two weeks of care), instituting case conferences for high risk patients, introducing disease-specific and/or risk-specific management plans, and trying out nurse-physician scripts to improve communication with patients' primary care physicians. Most of the change ideas came from the ReACH National Collaborative, which had extracted a set of "high leverage" improvement ideas from the evaluation of an Acute Care Hospitalization "Toolkit" developed as part of the CMS 7th Scope of Work (Delmarva Foundation for Medical Care & Visiting Nurse Service of New York, 2005). The toolkit included an inventory of effective practices based in part on synthesis of the available scientific literature on reducing hospitalization through improved patient management in the home.

Among the most useful strategies and tools cited by the respondents were:

- Instituting risk-appropriate care plans (6 respondents)
- Front-loading visits for high risk patients (6 respondents)
- Establishing patient emergency response plans (4 respondents)
- Introducing disease management tools (4 respondents)
- Using nurse-physician scripts and educational tools (3 respondents)

Generally, these change ideas were judged useful because they matched one of the priority areas outlined by ReACH (i.e., improving transitions, targeting interventions according to patients' risk, supporting effective care management and enhancing MD-home care communication); offered specific, easy to interpret suggestions for implementation; and/or corresponded to a perceived performance gap in the agency. For some agencies, the opportunity to try out a new practice was an important plus, while for others, compatibility with established agency practices was the primary consideration. Some would have liked additional sample tools from which to choose, including examples of patient emergency care plans, a greater selection of risk assessment tools, chronic disease pathways and staffing templates for frontloaded visits.

Respondents reported a variety of lessons learned from their early tests of change. Some observed that staff became more committed to the ReACH initiative when they had the opportunity to learn about proposed changes through the testing process and to provide feedback on specific strategies. Some became more aware of the already high demands on staff time and the need to tailor changes to account for resource constraints. Done carefully, these respondents concluded, testing could be a good way to involve staff and to sustain interest and commitment. Some respondents emphasized the value of starting small and fixing small scale mistakes before going agency wide, while others emphasized the importance of using a large enough population when testing a strategy to allow for generalizability. Overall, small scale testing was judged to be an effective way of preparing for larger scale change, especially with careful monitoring and associated adjustments to the testing effort.

Measurement Strategy

Measuring changes in care processes and patient outcomes in order to monitor agency progress over time is a key feature of the ReACH Collaborative. Each month each participating agency is asked to input data on seven measures for a minimum of 20 patient episodes. The data are entered on the ReACH Collaborative website, where an agency can instantly see a run chart that tracks its progress over time in comparison to the goals it set at baseline and the progress of all other agencies in the Collaborative (an aggregate measure). The measures include: percentage of patient episodes for which a risk assessment was conducted, percentage of "at risk" patients with a risk-appropriate care plan completed in 5 days, average number of clinical contacts a patient receives within the first 2 weeks of care, and hospitalization rate for the target population and for the agency as a whole.

Overall, ten of the respondents thought the ReACH monthly measurement data and reports were somewhat useful in guiding improvement efforts, while another seven found them very useful. The measurement data and reports were judged most useful because they:

- Benchmarked agency performance with national data (12 respondents)
- Provided necessary feedback on improvement activities (9 respondents)
- Guided improvement actions going forward (8 respondents)
- Gave immediate results (1 respondent)

Findings from High-Performing Agencies

Additional interviews with the four high-performing agencies revealed several factors contributing to their early success in reducing acute care hospitalizations. These agencies achieved successful staff buy-in at the beginning of the Collaborative through active communication and internal training. They credited their QIOs for providing a strong orientation and helpful information, and they attributed their success in part to the structure and approach of the ReACH Collaborative, with its emphasis on systematic improvement methods. Substantively, frontloading visits for high-risk patients was most often cited as key to reducing ACH. Perhaps the most outstanding feature of these high performing agencies was the active support of top leadership. With one exception (where there was a transition in agency directors), respondents described leadership as "very involved" and "supportive" of the project. For example, directors attended team meetings, participated in the project as team members and provided additional resources to the team when needed.

RECOMMENDATIONS

Respondents' suggestions for improving the ReACH Collaborative fell into three main categories:

1. Better preparing agencies to participate in the Collaborative by: streamlining the "Prework"/Planning Phase, providing simpler work instructions, and clarifying expectations regarding agency time and resource commitment necessary for effective implementation
2. Sharpening the focus on leadership and staffing issues at the agency level by emphasizing: the importance of high level commitment, investment in staff training at the beginning of the project, and ongoing efforts to gain staff buy-in and engagement
3. Providing more effective and efficient technical assistance at the local level by encouraging and equipping QIOs to: help agencies develop and implement data collection and management systems, offer more "best practice" improvement strategies, and organize information sharing among agencies with similar characteristics (e.g., agency size, population mix)

Wave II of ReACH, which started in October 2006, is incorporating many of these recommendations into the work plan, including:

1. Revised Planning Packet with simplified instructions, examples of key activities and responses to common questions
2. Revised Planning/Prework workshop for new agencies, providing a detailed description of activities, clear expectations for participation and recommendations for successful participation based on experiences of Wave I agencies
3. Additional Workshops by QIOs to review the Plannning/Prework activities in detail
4. One-to-One QIOs meetings with home health agency leaders to clearly define expectations for participation and address issues of leadership commitment and team responsibilities for ReACH
5. Mentoring of Wave II agencies, whereby Wave I agencies will participate in the local learning sessions as well as the monthly team conference calls and ReACH partnership calls, providing an opportunity for peer learning and direct sharing of best practices and agency-specific experiences for reducing acute care hospitalizations

CONCLUSION

As is common in many quality improvement initiatives across the health care system, ReACH agencies faced a variety of implementation challenges related to scarce staff resources, time constraints and competing priorities. Four months into the Collaborative most were in the process of addressing these challenges and reported that their efforts were yielding some success. A variety of factors–both internal and external to the agencies–were judged to facilitate participation in the ReACH Collaborative. Internally, strong leadership, as well as prior concern and/or experience in addressing acute care hospitalization, helped agencies successfully address the challenges involved in implementing the changes called for by ReACH. Externally, both ReACH project resources and QIO support were perceived as important factors contributing to successful involvement in the initiative.

Many agencies voiced concerns about the multiple causes of patient hospitalization, the limited sphere of home care influence and the limited ability of a home care agency acting alone to reduce hospital admissions. However, at the time of the interviews, the majority of ReACH participants had focused their efforts on internal processes and systems to effectively identify and manage patients at greatest risk of hospitalization. These included: implementing risk assessment procedures, introducing or increasing telemonitoring, frontloading visits, and instituting emergency care plans with patient-focused recommendations for those at greatest risk. Subsequently, several agencies have begun to work closely with hospital partners on strategies to improve patient transitions from hospital to home care, although the results of these interventions are not yet in.

Today virtually all home health agencies are familiar with the challenges of quality improvement and practice change. Outcomes Based Quality Improvement (OBQI) has become a byword of the home health care industry with the emergence of the CMS "Home Health Compare" website and its ten national OASIS-based indicators, the requirements of the two national home care accrediting bodies, and the growing impetus for quality improvement provided by the national network of QIOs and the new QIO-driven national Home Health Quality Improvement Campaign. Increasing financial pressure from the CMS prospective payment system to deliver care both effectively and economically and the impending arrival of a new pay-for-performance reimbursement system, which may include acute care hospitalization rates as one of its criteria for payment, also are affecting the industry.

Several barriers, however, have heightened the challenges of quality improvement in home care. These include relative isolation from mainstream academic and professional initiatives to establish national, evidence-based guidelines and standards (Feldman, Clark, & Bruno, 2006), lack of prior involvement in national "breakthrough" collaboratives and campaigns, as well as the relatively small size, flat administrative structure and lack of highly specialized quality improvement specialists in many agencies. A major premise of the ReACH design was that collaborative quality improvement with its formal structure, built-in technical assistance and sharing of problems and solutions would be especially well suited to compensating for the industry's isolation and scarcity of sophisticated quality improvement resources. Additional assumptions were that: (1) local technical assistance would expand access and improve sustainability of successful improvements; (2) collaboration with the QIOs would be the most powerful tool for disseminating quality improvement expertise at the local level; (3) ReACH technical assistance targeted primarily to QIOs would be critical to success of the effort; and (4) "multimodal" collaboration with a strong virtual component (i.e., list serves, web casts and web-based data collection) would significantly leverage the resources of both the national ReACH and the local QIO staff.

Although it would be premature to make a definitive judgment about the accuracy of these premises, the early evaluation results presented here suggest that the collaborative aspects of ReACH have been important in contributing to the successful implementation of the hospitalization initiative so far. In particular, the structure of the Collaborative and the tools and instructions it has developed have enabled agencies to experiment with mechanisms for systematically identifying patient risk and targeting clinical resources accordingly, a concept that underpins existing research on improving patient transitions but is quite new to the home care industry. The Collaborative also has provided participating agencies with a clear set of directives on systemic changes that must be implemented to successfully manage risk of hospitalization. Prime among these are improving care management and strengthening communication and coordination within the home care team and between the home care team and patients' physicians–practice improvements that have been the foundation of successful, rigorous transition research to date (Naylor, 2002, 2006; Naylor et al., 1999; Naylor et al., 2004; Phillips et al., 2004). Lastly, the cooperation between the national ReACH Project Staff and the QIOs participating in the first wave of the Collaborative has been a model of leveraged resources that has met with widespread approval of the participating ReACH agencies. Only time will tell, however, whether the broad recommendations provided and the extent of implementation achieved will result in significant reductions in patient hospitalization, which is a function of many complicated factors both within and outside the direct control of home care providers.

REFERENCES

Coleman, E., Parry, A., Chalmers, S., & Sung-Joon, M. (2006). The care transitions intervention: Results of a randomized controlled trial. *Archives of Internal Medicine, 166*, 1822-1828.

Delmarva Foundation for Medical Care. (2005). *Acute Care Hospitalization of Home Health Patients: Report of Analyses, Literature Review, and Technical Expert Panel.* Easton, Maryland: Unpublished.

Delmarva Foundation for Medical Care and Visiting Nurse Service of New York. (2005). *Reducing Acute Care Hospitalization* (Publication No. HH QIOSC 082008–001). Easton, MD: Unpublished.

Feldman, P.H., Clark, A., & Bruno, L. (2006). Advancing the agenda for home healthcare quality: Conference proceedings and findings. *Home Healthcare Nurse, 24*(5), 282-89.

Mistiaen, P., & Poot, E. (2006). Telephone follow-up initiated by a hospital based health professional, for post discharge problems in patients discharged from hospital to home. Cochrane Database of Systematic Review. Cochrane Library, Issue 4. Art. No.: CD004510. DOI: 10. 1002/14651858.CD004510.pub3.

Naylor, M.D. (2002). Transitional care of older adults. *Annual Review of Nursing Research, 20*, 127-47.

Naylor, M.D. (2006). Transitional care: A critical dimension of the home healthcare quality agenda. *Journal for Healthcare Quality, 28*(1), 48-54.

Naylor, M.D., Brooten, D., Campbell, R., Jacobsen, B.S., Mezey, M.D., Pauly, M.V., & Schwartz, J.S. (1999). Comprehensive discharge planning and home follow-up of hospitalized elders: A randomized clinical trial. *Journal of the American Medical Association, 281*(7), 613-20.

Naylor, M.D., Brooten, D.A., Campbell, R., Maislin, G., McCauley, K.M., & Schwartz, J.S. (2004). Transitional care of older adults hospitalized with heart failure: A randomized, controlled trial. *Journal of the American Geriatrics Society, 52*(5), 675-84. Erratum in: *Journal of the American Geriatrics Society* (2004), *52*(7), 1228.

Phillips, C.O., Wright, S.M., Kern, D.E., Singa, R.M., Sheppard, S., & Rubin, H.R. (2004). Comprehensive discharge planning with post-discharge support for older patients with congestive heart failure: A meta-analysis. *Journal of the American Medical Association, 291*(11), 1358-67.

Rosati, R.J., Huang, L., Navaie-Waliser, M., Feldman, & P.H. (2003). Risk factors for repeated hospitalization among home healthcare recipients. *Journal of Healthcare Quality, 25*(2), 38-45.

World Health Organization. (2005). *Do current discharge arrangements from inpatient hospital care for the elderly reduce readmission rates, the length of inpatient stay or mortality, or improve health status?* Regional Office for Europe's Health Evidence Network [HEN].

doi:10.1300/J027v26n04_08

A Research and Policy Agenda
for Transitions from Nursing Homes to Home

Peter A. Boling, MD
Pamela Parsons, PhD, RN

SUMMARY. More than 1 million adults make the transition from nursing homes to the community every year, often using formal health services including Medicare Part A skilled home health care. Although the need for discharge planning is well described, and the risks associated with care transitions are increasingly recognized, there is very limited information about the process and outcomes as patients move from nursing home to home. This paper reviews pertinent published data and health services research as background information and outlines a research agenda for studying these important transitions. doi:10.1300/J027v26n04_09 *[Article copies available for a fee from The Haworth Document Delivery Service: 1-800-HAWORTH. E-mail address: <docdelivery@haworthpress.com> Website: <http://www.HaworthPress.com> © 2007 by The Haworth Press, Inc. All rights reserved.]*

KEYWORDS. Nursing homes, home care services, care transitions

---

Peter A. Boling is Professor, Department of Medicine, Virginia Commonwealth University, PO Box 980102, Richmond, VA 23298 (E-mail: pboling@vcu.edu).

Pamela Parsons is Assistant Professor, Department of Medicine, Virginia Commonwealth University, PO Box 980102, Richmond, VA 23298 (E-mail: pparsons@vcu.edu).

[Haworth co-indexing entry note]: "A Research and Policy Agenda for Transitions from Nursing Homes to Home." Boling, Peter A. and Pamela Parsons. Co-published simultaneously in *Home Health Care Services Quarterly®* (The Haworth Press, Inc.) Vol. 26, No. 4, 2007, pp. 121-131; and: *Charting a Course for High Quality Care Transitions* (ed: Eric A. Coleman) The Haworth Press, Inc. 2007, pp. 121-131. Single or multiple copies of this article are available for a fee from The Haworth Document Delivery Service [1-800-HAWORTH, 9:00 a.m. - 5:00 p.m. (EST). E-mail address: docdelivery@haworthpress.com].

INTRODUCTION

A rapid upsurge occurred in use of Medicare post-acute care after prospective payment changed hospital incentives in 1984. Revisions in payment models for home health and nursing home care followed, recently shifting to accommodate these post-acute care utilization patterns. Unfortunately, although transitions and movement through other venues of health care delivery (e.g., hospital discharges) have received research and policy attention nursing home discharges to home and the key role of home health care in this context continue to exist as the "neglected stepchild" of care transitions.

In 2003, there were approximately 2.34 million Medicare skilled nursing home admissions with Medicare covering on average 25 days of care at a daily rate of $434 (Health Care Financing Review, 2005). The principal diagnoses were heterogeneous, as with all Medicare Part A services, with a strong influence from cardiovascular ailments. In 1997, of 2.1 million nursing home discharges, most died or went to the hospital; with no clear data regarding the number that discharge from nursing home to home with home care (Gabrel, 2000). This paper focuses on the time following discharge from Medicare Part A skilled nursing home care to other community living settings. We searched the medical literature for articles that inform attempts to improve the quality of care following these transitions and suggest research opportunities to improve the delivery of health services during this process.

Current Care Environment

To date, patterns of movement through post-acute care (PAC) have been studied at the macro level. Using the 1994 National Long Term Care Survey Murtaugh (2002) found that between 1992 and 1994, 18 percent of elders were admitted to or discharged from a study setting, and 22 percent subsequently used health services of some type (rehabilitation hospital, nursing home, or home health care). Analysis of federal utilization data from the mid-1990's suggests that many factors influence pathways through post-acute care, including practice style, supply, and local regulation (Kane, Lin & Blewett, 2002). Usage patterns appeared to follow financial incentives after the 1997 Balanced Budget Act, yet analysis of large databases suggests that there is considerable opportunity for substitution between types of post-acute care (inpatient rehabilitation, skilled nursing home, and skilled home health care) (Lin et al., 2006).

On a positive note, despite the recent incentive changes there has been no documented increased risk of death or decline in eventual discharge home from nursing homes (Wodchis, Fries & Hirth, 2004). However, information available regarding individual care settings (hospital, nursing home and home health care) raises alarming concern about patient safety during chronic care episodes. Frequent re-hospitalization during post-acute care demonstrates instability and indicates suboptimal care process. Patients newly enrolled in Medicare skilled home health care services have a high risk-adjusted hospitalization rate (nationally over 30 percent) within the first 60 days of Medicare Part A home health care (Rollow et al., 2006). Similarly high rates of hospital use are seen in nursing home populations and in life care communities, even when geriatric care models are employed that can produce better results (Phillips et al., 2000). The transition from nursing home to home, where care has been within a monitored system with 24-hour nursing and care-giving support to the independent environment of the home setting, represents one of the periods of highest risk for error and poor outcomes.

The authors' observations from caring for thousands of patients during the past 8 years as they moved through acute and post-acute care in Richmond, Virginia lend personal credence to the difficulties encountered in maintaining high quality, safe transitions during this phase. Due in part to low historical service utilization, the Richmond area lacks Medicare risk contracts and the health care financing environment is shaped by Medicare Part A. Patients typically come to nursing homes from hospitals with limited, incomplete or fragmentary clinical information about the hospital course and nominal attempts at medication reconciliation that sometimes appear credible and are often erroneous. Care plans are re-created at the nursing home where most patients stay for fewer than 21 days (the point at which Medicare Part A requires a $119 daily co-payment). Often the primary care physician has not heard about the hospital admission that started the care episode or the nursing home admission. The quality of nursing home discharge planning is variable, and institutional providers depend on family caregivers to patch the quilt together. When patients transition home from nursing homes, there is little or no communication about clinical details to home health agencies or physicians responsible for ongoing care. This risky environment has evolved and persists despite recent emphasis on patient safety and is aggravated by the Health Care Portability and Accountability Act which leads hospital-based providers to withhold health care information from those responsible for post-acute care.

Nursing Home Population and Discharges to Home

To grasp the needs of the nursing home patient that may be transitioning to home, we must first understand the resident population. Some residents have a good prognosis and are recovering from an acute problem, such as elective surgery; others are on a downward health and functional trajectory, and some of them moved to the nursing home from other settings with formal support services, such as assisted living facilities (ALF).

Patients moving to nursing homes from assisted living facilities (ALFs) are usually declining. A recent literature review on ALFs found several large surveys that had varied methods and rigor but also generally consistent findings that individuals moving from ALFs to nursing homes are less likely to successfully return home. In ALFs, physical dependency and cognitive impairment (34 to 52 percent) are common problems, 28 percent die in the ALF, 11 to 18 percent are discharged to hospital, and 33 to 36 percent are discharged to nursing home for health reasons (Golant, 2004). ALFs are often a way station for individuals on a downward health trajectory who do not require the full range of nursing home services at the time of ALF enrollment and stay an average of 3.5 years (Phillips et al., 2003) before dying or moving to a higher level of care. Most people who move from ALFs to nursing homes do so because of declining health and functional status (Phillips et al, 2003) rather than dementia and behavioral issues (Rosenberg et al, 2006).

An excellent analysis by the Congressional Budget Office (High-Cost Medicare Beneficiaries, Congressional Budget Office Report, 2005) shows that high-cost outliers with multiple health problems tend to be recurrent heavy users of Medicare resources, such as nursing home, at many points over a five-year interval. Comparing site of death for all US Medicare Part A nursing home residents who died in 2001, Levy and colleagues (2004) found greater age and functional impairment associated with death in nursing homes, as expected. However, comparing outcomes by state, there was as much as 4-fold variation in the likelihood that an individual would die in the hospital rather than the nursing home.

The literature shows that individual characteristics predict PAC outcomes. Functional status variables identify support needs of hospital patients at discharge. Older adults discharged home from the hospital to live alone are at high risk of poor outcomes. One might expect that particular attention would be paid to people making that transition a few weeks later after a nursing home stay. Multiple studies have shown that active therapy in the nursing home setting increases the likelihood of successful discharge to home both for hip fractures and other conditions again this is no surprise and may incorporate selection bias since those that receive active therapy in the nursing home likely have more rehabilitative potential (Harada, Chun, Chiu & Pakalniskis, 2000 and Arling, Williams & Kopp, 2000). While intuitively obvious, these findings could be part of a framework to promote safer care processes.

Role of Discharge Planning

Patients with advanced chronic illness and a history of recurrent service utilization that suggests a declining health trajectory need more comprehensive planning. One consideration is whether care plans are made by regular day staff or by those covering evenings, nights, and weekends. Factors rated highly by both nursing home medical directors and nursing home staff as predictors of excess hospitalization included lack of information about patients' problems and lack of familiarity with patients on the part of physicians taking after-hours call (Buchanan et al., 2006).

Medication-related problems deserve special note. These are one of the common mechanisms for adverse outcomes such as re-hospitalization and disability (Forster et al., 2003). Following discharge from hospital to community, several studies have now found discrepancies in the care plan including medications; in one study, 14 percent of patients had discrepancies and those with discrepancies were more than twice as likely to be re-hospitalized within 30 days (Coleman et al., 2005). There are no studies to confirm this observation in the context of nursing home discharges; compared with hospitals, the slower pace of nursing home care allows more time for planning, but the same problems may exist. Even though medication reconciliation is a focal point for JCAHO certification, the extent to which this policy is implemented or effectively evaluated when patients move from hospitals into post-acute care remains problematic.

Some groundwork for improved nursing home discharge planning is already laid. The process is not unique and existing templates that describe discharge planning in other settings, such as the hospital, could arguably also be applied to nursing home discharges (Potthof, Kane & Franco, 1997). As this area receives more attention, it is important to adopt a patient-centered approach to planning various phases of post-acute care as noted by Parry and colleagues (2003). This sound premise places the focus where it should be.

Role of Care Providers

There are published examples of improved processes that deliver better post-discharge outcomes. An intervention to empower patients and caregivers and enable better post-hospital transitional care reduced the likelihood of re-hospitalization from home within 30, 90, or 180 days, and like several other recent post-acute care models reduced rate of hospitalization by about 50 percent (Coleman et al, 2004). Similarly, in the nursing home setting, active case management directed primarily by advance practice nurses can improve utilization patterns and control acute care costs without sacrificing quality, measured by major endpoints such as mortality (Kane, Flood, Bershadsky, Keckhafer, 2004). In a small randomized controlled trial, researchers have studied one model of augmented discharge planning to improve return to the community after a nursing home stay with relatively modest effects but risk of Type II error due to the small study size (Newcomer, Kang & Graham, 2006; Graham, Anderson, & Newcomer, 2005).

Role of Home Care

Referrals to home care following nursing home care should include therapy programs for those with better prognoses. Continued physical therapy at home following discharge from inpatient rehabilitation units has been shown to confer additional benefit (Intrator & Berg, 1998). Increasing cost pressures invite more intense scrutiny of care processes for efficiency and quality, and federal policy-makers have questioned the relative value of home care leading to reduced funding and fewer services. A recent review criticized home care studies for inconsistently measuring indirect costs (Ramosa, Ferraz & Sesso, 2004). In planning future analyses we should avoid holding home care to a higher standard of proof than other venues.

Role of Family and Caregivers

While home-based care certainly rests heavily on the shoulders of lay caregivers, institutional care involves similar elements; family caregivers spend much time visiting during hospital or nursing home care, and addressing complex issues that are critical to future care plans, such as making provisions for support (feeding, bathing, grooming); participating in medical decision-making; working on insurance coverage, financing, and social networks; and visiting alternate institutional care settings.

A RESEARCH AGENDA AND POLICY REFORM
FOR NURSING HOME DISCHARGES TO HOME

The Deficit Reduction Act (DRA) of 2005 was signed into law on February 8, 2006; Section 8 mandates post-acute care payment reform and this requirement is aligned with the stated CMS vision for post-acute care reform. The PAC Reform Plan centers on Post–Acute Care Payment Systems and Assessment Instruments, and directly addresses the needs of chronically ill elders. It also provides a guiding framework for a research agenda for this vulnerable population (Policy Council Document, Post-Acute Care Reform Plan, 2006).

Currently, Medicare's policies and reimbursement have focused on phases of illness, defined by site of service, rather than specific characteristics and care needs of the individual who moves across settings. CMS now operates four separate prospective payment systems for each PAC provider setting, using standardized approaches for quality assessment and control, and to determine payment. The systems are individualized to each site of service; for example, skilled nursing facilities use the Minimum Data Set (MDS) and certified home health agencies use the Outcome and Assessment Information Set (OASIS). These data systems share several domains (e.g., cognition, affective, behavioral, physiologic, and functional) but use different forms and formats, ask questions in different ways, store data in separate databases and collect information at varied time intervals. Some outcomes and quality indicators are similar, but standardization across settings is lacking. For example, hospitals and home health agencies track emergency room use as an outcome indicator, but nursing homes do not.

The first step in quality improvement and policy change is measurement. As stated by Coleman and Berenson (2004) we need better information to develop systems of care. Where do these people go? What formal health care services do they receive? Do they use acute care again, and if so, how soon after the transition? What are their health outcomes and mortality rates? Once we have basic service utilization data, the extensive clinical data that are gathered in nursing homes should enable us to dissect the relative contributions and interactions of many factors associated with utilization patterns and outcomes. The Minimum Data Set provides patient-level characteristics that can be combined with facility data (OSCAR, nursing home regulatory surveys), and patient outcomes in cross-level analyses (Goodman P, 2002). We should be able to identify groups of patients who are at particularly high risk of poor outcomes, and we should be able to improve nursing home care processes using these analyses. For example, care planning using clinical and administrative data obtained on admission can anticipate post-discharge needs of nursing home patients (Murtaugh et al., 1994).

When patients are discharged to the community from nursing homes without formal Medicare Part A skilled home care we have no established means to track health outcomes, but for those receiving skilled home care an interesting albeit complex analysis could be organized by combining MDS data with OASIS data to describe the trajectory as individuals successively move through domains in the post-acute care service spectrum.

Reliable data are essential. In this regard, home care has been helped by implementation of the Outcomes and Assessment Information Set (OASIS), though agency training in use of this tool has varied. Additional work remains to reconcile measurements made using the nursing home Minimum Data Set with OASIS items. OASIS and MDS were designed for different purposes and are not interchangeable. They are also deeply imbedded in business, operational and quality measurement systems that involve hundreds of billions of dollars, hundreds of thousands of providers and tens of thousands of organizations annually.

It would be useful to conduct prospective studies that examine specific issues such as medication reconciliation and medication errors following transitions from nursing home to home, as have been done in the hospital-to-home transition, and to compare the pattern across all acute care and post-acute care settings.

Another untested hypothesis is that broader access to a reliable electronic health record would prevent many of the problems that now arise from discontinuities as patients with advanced chronic illness move through post-acute care settings.

Compelling data (High-Cost Medicare Beneficiaries, Congressional Budget office, 2005) show that patients with extensive co-morbidity have persistent high utilization patterns over most of a five-year period. Yet the continuum of geriatric care is a concept in name only for most communities and most patients. Active medical care management has been shown to stabilize high-risk patients following hospital discharge (Naylor et al., 1999) and in nursing homes (Kane et al., 2004). Similar approaches could work following nursing home discharge, but are untested. Care models exist that provide longitudinal services across settings, but most are time-limited. Studies may show that relatively intensive case management strategies have diminishing returns as the interval following an acute problem lengthens and patients stabilize. With that cautionary note, the patient-centered framework tempts us to favor models that afford continuity of care throughout the concluding years for frail and vulnerable individuals and their families. The trade-off between cost and quality is something that can and should be measured. Meanwhile, this patient-centered, continuity-oriented approach is the one that we follow in Richmond, Virginia as we observe the inexorably rising and increasingly urgent demand for a health care system that addresses population needs.

CONCLUSION

CMS and Congress have now recognized the need to remedy the imploding care matrix that exists for the chronically ill elderly: one mandate of the PAC Reform Plan is creation of a standardized assessment and information tool that will follow patients across the care continuum. In addition demonstration projects that will include evaluation of proposed financing and assessment measures are due to begin in 2008. We are hopeful, that with a carefully outlined research agenda and the support of public policy we can make positive steps towards improving quality in health transitions for the generation to come.

REFERENCES

Arling G, Williams AR, & Kopp D. (2000).Therapy use and discharge outcomes for elderly nursing home residents. *Gerontologist, 40*(5), 587-95.

Buchanan JL, Murkofsky RL, O'Malley AJ, Karon SL, Zimmerman D, Caudry DJ & Marcantonio ER. (2006). Nursing home capabilities and decisions to hospitalize: A survey of medical directors and directors of nursing. *Journal of the American Geriatrics Society, 54*, 458-465.

Coleman, EA, & Berenson, RN (2004). Lost in transition: challenges and opportunites in moving patients between health care settings *Annals of Internal Medicine, 41*(7), 533-536.

Coleman EA, MD, Smith JD, Raha D, & Min SJ. (2005).Post hospital medication discrepancies: Prevalence and contributing factors. *Archives of Internal Medicine,165*, 1842-1847.

Forster AJ, Murff HJ, Peterson JF, Gandhi TK, & Bates DW. (2003)The incidence and severity of adverse events affecting patients after discharge from the hospital. *Annals of Internal* Medicine*, 138*, 161-167.

Fortinsky, RH, Covinsky KE, Palmer, RM & Landefedl, CS. (1999). Effects of functional status changes before and during hospitalization and nursing home admission of older adults. *Journal of Gerontology A Biological Science and Medical Science, 54*(10), M521-526.

Gabrel, CS. (2000). Characteristics of elderly nursing home current residents and discharges: Data from from the 1997 National Nursing Home Survey. *Adv Data. Apr 25*(312), 1-15.

Golant SM.(2004). Do impaired older persons with health care needs occupy U.S. assisted living Facilities: An analysis of six national studies: *Journal of Gerontology, 59B*(2), S68-S79.

Goodman, PS (2000). Missing organizational linkages: Tools for cross-level research. Thousand Oaks, CA: Foundations for Organizational Science, Sage Publications, Inc.

Graham, C, Anderson, L, & Newcomer R (2005). Nursing home transition; Providing assistance to caregivers in transition program. *Lippincott's Case Management, 10*(2), 93-101.

Harada, ND, Chun, A, Chiu, V. & Pakalniskis, A. (2000). Patterns of rehabilitation utilization after hip fracture in acute hospitals and skilled nursing facilities *Medical Care, 38*(11), 1119-1130.

Health Care Financing Review. Medicare and Medicaid Statistical Supplement, 2005: 120-125.

High-cost Medicare Beneficiaries. Congressional Budget Office (May, 2005).

Intrator, O, & Berg K. (1998). Benefits of home health care after inpatient rehabilitation for hip fracture: Health service use by Medicare beneficiaries, 1987-1992. *Archives of Physical Rehabilitation, 79*(10), 1195-1199.

Kane, RL , Lin, WC & Blewett, LA (2002). Geographic variation in the use of post-acute care. *Health Services Research, 37*(3), 667-682.

Kane R, Flood S, Bershadsky, B, & Keckhafer, G. (2004). Effect of an innovative Medicare managed care program on the quality of care for nursing home residents. Gerontologist, *44*(1), 95-103.

Levy, CR, Fish R, & Kramer, AM (2004). Site of death in the hospital versus nursing home of Medicare skilled nursing facility residents admitted under Medicare's Part A benefit. *Journal of the American Geriatrics Society, 52*, 1247-1254.

Lin, WC, Kane RL, Mehr, DR., Madsen, RW, & Petroski, GF (2006). Changes in the use of postacute care during the initial Medicare payment reforms. *Health Services Research, 41*(4 Pt 1), 1338-1356.

Mahoney, JE, Eisner, J, Havighurst, T Gray, S, & Palta, M (2000). Problems of older adults living alone after hospitalization. *Journal of General Internal Medicine, 15*(9), 673-674.

Murtaugh, CM. (1994). Discharge planning in nursing homes. *Health Services Research, 28*(6), 751-769.

Murtaugh, CM, & Litke, A. (2002). Transitions through postacute and long-term care settings: Patterns of use and outcomes for a national cohort of elders. *Medical Care, 40*(3), 227-236.

Naylor, MD, Brooten, D, Campbell, R., Jacobsen, BS, Mezey, MD, Pauly, MV, & Schwartz, JS. Comprehensive discharge planning and home care follow-up of hospitalized elders. *Journal of the American Medical Association, 281*(7), 613-620.

Newcomer, R, Kang, T & Graham, C. (2006). Outcomes in a nursing home transition case-management program targeting new admissions. *Gerontologist, 46*(3), 385-390.

Parry, C, Coleman, EA, Smith, JD, Frank, J, & Kramer, AM. (2003). The care transitions Intervention: A patient-centered approach to ensuring effective transfers between sites of geriatric care. *Home Health Care Services Quarterly, 20*(30), 1-17.

Phillips, CD, Munoz, Y, Sherman, M, Rose, M, Spector, W, & Hawes, C. (2003). Effects of facility characteristics on departures from assisted living: Results from a national study. *Gerontologist, 43*, 690-696.

Phillips, VL, Paul, W, Becker, ER, Osterweil, D, & Ouslander, JG (2000). Health care utilization by old-old long-term care facility residents how do Medicare fee-for-service and capitation rates compare? *Journal of the American Geriatrics Society, 48*(10), 1330-1336.

Policy Council Document, Post-Acute Care Reform Plan, 2006. http://www.cms. hhs.gov/ QualityInitiativesGenInfo/downloads/QualityPACFullReport.pdf.

Potthoff, S, Kane, RL, & Franco, SJ. (1997). Improving hospital discharge planning for elderly patients. *Health Care Financing Review, 19*(2), 47-72.

Ramosa, MLT, Ferraz, MB & Sesso R. (2004). Critical appraisal of published economic evaluations of home care for the elderly. *Archives of Gerontology and Geriatrics, 39*, 255-267.

Rosenberg, PB, Mielke, MM, Samus, QM, Rosenblatt, A, Baker, A, Brandt, J, Rabins, PV & Lyketsos, CG. (2006). Transition to nursing home from assisted living is not associated with dementia or dementia-related problem behaviors. *Journal of the American Medical Directors Association, 7*, 73-78.

Rollow, W, Lied, TR, McGann, P, Poywer, J, LaVole, L, Kambie, RT, Bratzler, DW, Ma, A, Huff, ED, & Ramunno, LD (2006). Assessment of the Medicare quality improvement organization program. *Annals of Internal Medicine, 145*, 342-353.

Wodchis, WP, Fries, BF, & Hirth, RA (2004). The effect of Medicare's prospective payment System on discharge outcomes of skilled nursing facility residents. *Inquiry, 41*(4), 418-434.

doi:10.1300/J027v26n04_09

Index